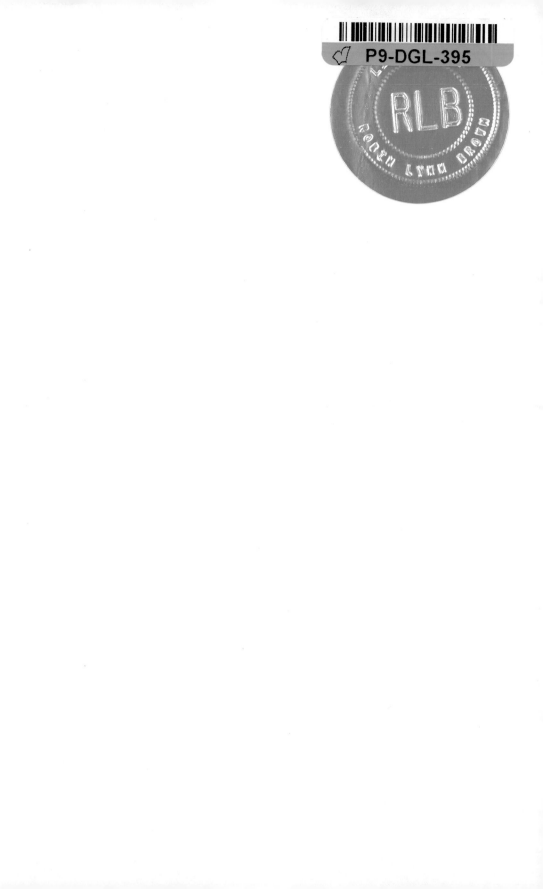

DEMENTIA AND MEMORY

To Moose and Bogey,
David and Beverley,
and Natalie

"Life is so time-consuming
But worth every second."
SBNT

Dementia and Memory
A Handbook for Students and Professionals

PROFESSOR SIMON B. N. THOMPSON
Neuropsychology Assessment & Consultancy, Portsmouth, UK

ASHGATE

Published by
Ashgate Publishing Limited
Gower House
Croft Road
Aldershot
Hampshire GU11 3HR
England

Ashgate Publishing Company
Suite 420
101 Cherry Street
Burlington, VT 05401-4405
USA

Ashgate website: http://www.ashgate.com

British Library Cataloguing in Publication Data
Thompson, Simon B. N.
   Dementia and memory : a handbook for students and
   professionals
   1.Dementia 2.Memory disorders in old age
   I.Title
   616.8'3

Library of Congress Cataloging-in-Publication Data
Thompson, Simon B. N.
   Dementia and memory : a handbook for students and professionals / by Simon B. N. Thompson.
          p. cm.
   Includes bibliographical references and index.
   ISBN 0-7546-4633-5
   1. Memory disorders in old age--Handbooks, manuals, etc. 2. Dementia--Handbooks, manuals, etc. I. Title

   RC394.M46T365 2006
   616.8'3--dc22

                                                      2006003913

ISBN-10: 0 7546 4633 5
ISBN-13: 978 0 7546 4633 4

Printed and bound in Great Britain by Antony Rowe Ltd, Chippenham, Wiltshire.

Contents

List of Figures		*ix*
List of Tables		*xi*
Preface		*xiii*
Acknowledgements		*xv*
Introduction		*xvii*

PART I   DEFINING DEMENTIA AND MEMORY

1.   Introduction to Dementia   3

     Background   3
     Normal Ageing   3
     Physical and Psychological Problems of Ageing   7
     Normal Memory   8
     Memory and Dementia   10
     Anxiety and Dementia   14
     Ageism   15
     Further Reading   17

2.   Definition of Dementia   19

     Alzheimer's Disease   20
     Vascular Dementia   30
     Subcortical Arteriosclerotic Encephalopathy   34
     Pick's Disease   34
     Parkinson's Disease   35
     Huntington's Disease   36
     Creutzfeldt-Jakob Disease   38
     Multiple Sclerosis   40
     Motor Neurone Disease   41
     Dementia Pugilistica   42
     Pseudodementia   43
     Korsakoff's Psychosis   47
     Habit-forming Drugs and Toxins   49
     Differential Diagnosis   49
     Further Reading   51

3. Memory Disorders   53

    Intact Memory   53
    Types of Memory Disorders   54
    Memory Problems Associated with Dementia   55
    Further Reading   56

4. Learning Disability and Dementia   57

    Definition of 'Learning Disability'   57
    Definition of Down's Syndrome   57
    Link between Down's Syndrome and Alzheimer's Disease   58
    Difficulties in Identifying Dementia   59
    Social and Cultural Differences   61
    Social Rejection   63
    Further Reading   64

PART II COPING WITH MEMORY PROBLEMS

5. How to Treat Memory Problems   69

    External Aids and Tips   70
    Internal Strategies   71
    Teaching Memory Strategies to Others   74
    Further Reading   76

6. Advanced Memory Strategies   79

    Key Points in Helping People to Learn Strategies   79
    Remembering Complex Number Sequences   81
    Further Reading   82

7. Case Studies on Memory   83

    Memory Clinics   83

PART III COPING WITH DEMENTIA

8. How to Assess Dementia   91

    Taking Histories   91
    Assessing Functions in People with Dementia   91
    Assessing Memory   95
    Assessing Cognitive Abilities   96

Monitoring Behaviour 97
Methodological Considerations and Applicability of Tests 100
Some Conclusions about Assessment 101
Summary of Functions that should be Assessed 102
Further Reading 104

9. How to Cope with Dementia 107

Medical Treatment of Dementia 107
Offering Patients a Whole Package of Care 109
Reality Orientation 109
Further Reading 110

10. How to Manage Dementia 111
Psychological and Social Management of Dementia 111
Using Progressive Muscle Relaxation 112
Further Reading 115

11. Case Studies on Dementia 117

Clinical Trials 117
Working Memory in Alzheimer's Disease 118
Biochemical and Anatomical Studies of Dementia 121
Psychological Stress in Caregivers 122
Early Onset Dementia Clinics 122
Further Reading 126

12. Case Studies on Dementia and Learning Disability 127

People with Learning Disabilities and Dementia 127
Identifying Dementia in People with Down's Syndrome 128
Cognitive Decline with Age in Down's Syndrome 138
Central Executive System, Dementia and Learning
  Disability 141
Dementia and the Central Executive System 143
Discussion 155
Conclusions about Studies on Learning Disabilities
  and Dementia 160
Further Reading 160

13. Future Directions for People with Dementia 161

Screening Older People for Dementia 161
Genetic Link with Dementia 165

Medical Treatment for Alzheimer's Disease 166
Redefining Dementia 167
Further Reading 169

Test Your Long-term Memory 171
Section 1: Choice of Statements 171
Section 2: Supplementary Questions 178
Section 3: Answers 180
Glossary of Terms 183
Useful Journals and Magazines 191
Bibliography 193
Index 231

List of Figures

Figure 1.1   Depression and Dementia Compared   10

Figure 1.2   Similarities and Differences between Dementia and Other Problems   15

Figure 2.1   Schematic based on Baddeley's (1992) Working Memory Model   28

Figure 5.1   Using Word Association   76

Figure 7.1   Demographic Data (NART = National Adult Reading Test, an Estimate of Pre-morbid Intelligence or 'IQ')   86

Figure 7.2   Visual Memory Improvements   87

Figure 7.3   Verbal Memory Improvements   87

Figure 7.4   Pre and Post Anxiety and Depression Scores   88

Figure 8.1   Guidelines for a Structured Review   92

Figure 8.2   Personal History   93

Figure 8.3   Orientation Questions   94

Figure 8.4   The A-B-C Chart   97

Figure 8.5   Interval Sampling Record   98

Figure 8.6   Event Sampling Record   99

Figure 11.1   Schematic based on Baddeley's (1992) Working Memory Model   119

Figure 12.1   Client's Biographical Details   132

Figure 12.2   Anxiety and Depression Scale based on HADS   136

Figure 12.3   Clients'/Relatives' Consent Form   139

Figure 12.4   Schematic based on Baddeley's (1992) Working Memory Model   146

Figure 13.1   Percentage of People requiring Psychological Help   162

Figure 13.2   Percentage of People not requiring Psychological Help   163

Figure 13.3   Reasons for Psychological Help   164

List of Tables

Table 7.1   Demographic Data (NART = National Adult
             Reading Test, an Estimate of Pre-morbid
             Intelligence or 'IQ')   86
Table 12.1   Group 1: Summary of HSSA and WAIS-R
             Results   149
Table 12.2   Group 2: Summary of HSSA and WAIS-R
             Results   151
Table 12.3   Group 1: Comparison of Test Measures
             between Assessments 1 and 2   152
Table 12.4   Group 1: Comparison of Test Measures
             between Assessments 1 and 2 Controlling for
             'Anxiety' and 'Depression'   152
Table 12.5   Group 2: Comparison of Test Measures
             between Assessments 1 and 2   153
Table 12.6   Group 2: Comparison of Test Measures
             between Assessments 1 and 2 Controlling for
             'Anxiety' and 'Depression'   154
Table 12.7   Partial Correlation Coefficients for Group 1
             before and after Controlling for 'Anxiety' and
             'Depression'   154

Preface

The book is divided into three parts. Part I defines the various types of dementia within the context of ageing and abnormal ageing. The importance of memory and dementia is explained. Chapter 1 provides the reader with an overview of dementia that is designed to enlighten both the uninformed as well as the informed carer, therapist and clinician. The importance of recognising physical and psychological problems related to ageing is highlighted. Normal memory and memory functioning in dementia is presented as well as the problem of anxiety and dementia. The subject of ageism is discussed from several standpoints, together with some recommendations for good practice in the care of older people.

Chapter 2 defines the various types of dementias, distinguishing vascular from non-vascular types, and discusses the problems of differentiating dementia from depression in diagnosis. The causes and progress of each type of dementia are discussed. Chapter 3 presents memory disorders and how memory is affected by dementia. Chapter 4 is a specialist chapter on dementia and people with learning disabilities. The difficulty in identifying dementia in this population is presented, and the controversial topics of social and cultural differences and social rejection are discussed and evaluated.

Part II presents ways of coping with memory problems, discussing ways of assessing, treating and managing them. In Chapter 5, practical ways of treating memory problems are presented. Chapter 6 discusses how advanced strategies benefit people with memory problems. In Chapter 7, case studies on memory are presented and discussed.

In Part III, Chapters 8-13 are concerned with coping with dementia. Chapter 8 considers how dementia is assessed; in Chapter 9, various treatment options are discussed. The management of dementia is presented in Chapter 10 together with helpful suggestions.

In Chapters 11 and 12, case studies are discussed on dementia and learning disability, respectively. Finally, Chapter 13 presents future directions for helping people with dementia including work on genetics and medical treatment.

A test for long-term memory is included at the end of this book, divided into different decades to enable people to test people of different ages. Also included, is a list of useful journals and magazines for reference and a comprehensive bibliography, glossary and index.

Acknowledgements

Most people have at some time forgotten something. When it becomes important to remember a fact or where an object has been put, it becomes a frustration when the fact is forgotten or when the object is not found. Most of us have had a close relative who is in their sixties or older, or know of someone of a similar age. Some know the problems that can be related to age; others will know of the problems related to abnormal ageing, and most of us will experience ageing ourselves in time to come.

Many of us will have also used a derogatory term about an older person or know an ageist joke. The standpoint changes when the joke-teller eventually becomes the subject of the joke. For all of these reasons, it is helpful to look objectively and practically at the ageing process and how abnormal conditions, such as dementia, can affect us. By examining these processes, we will gain a better understanding and, hopefully, a more sympathetic approach to older people and those who have dementia and memory problems.

This book is inspired by my grandmother, an incredibly kind and intelligent lady. Fortunately, she maintained a remarkable memory all through her 94 years. Her humbleness and ability to examine opinion from others impressed me greatly.

I am grateful to several people who have helped me in my various professional pursuits: Dr Nigel North and Professor Narinder Kapur, and earlier in my career, Professor John MacDonald and Mr Mike Coleman. Latterly, I have benefited from reading the insights of established workers in the fields of dementia and neuropsychology, such as Robin Morris, Muriel Lezak, William Lishman, Helen Evenhuis, Barbara Wilson and in memory work, Alan Baddeley. This list is not exhaustive but represents some important contributions to psychology. It has also influenced the direction of my work, for which I am most grateful.

I would also like to thank Laura Sanger and Sarah Hardy for their support in the past; my parents for their continued support, my brother and Natalie for their encouragement and my colleagues and patients, who have made all this possible for me.

Simon B.N. Thompson
Portsmouth

Introduction

Dementia is a frightening and common 'illness'. The numbers of older people are steadily increasing, together with the demands on services, whether from relatives or paid staff. Part of this picture are older people with learning disabilities, who are also competing for existing services – some similar and some different – according to their own needs. This global picture of a growing mass of older people can be overwhelming. Unless we begin to put in place further services for the care of these people, we will be overwhelmed before we know it.

Putting in place appropriate services to provide for older people requires special skills. An appreciation of the concerns of older people is of paramount importance, and any changes in care patterns should be made in consultation with both the person who has dementia and the carer. Advocates can be invaluable in assisting in the provision of specialised care to individuals with dementia, whose needs may be numerous and varied. It should also be remembered that the management of dementia often takes place in the person's home.

Our attitude is sometimes influenced by the concept and terminology used when 'treating a patient with dementia', instead of 'caring for a person with dementia'. This is very important, as many interventions will involve long-term management or coping strategies rather than treatment. Dementia is often irreversible; approaches should focus more on improving quality of life, rather than treatment and cure.

Involving family and friends and setting up appropriate services is very important in enhancing the welfare and everyday functioning of the patient. Therefore, we should be looking towards improving living environments and community services, instead of hospital-based outreach facilities. The older population is on the increase, and we must be ready to provide adequate and appropriate facilities for them.

"Memory" has been defined in many ways. 'It is the faculty by which things are recalled to or kept in the mind; ...' (Thompson, 1995t, p.850). It is complicated by its various processes and hence it is difficult to study and sometimes difficult to treat when it goes wrong.

Memory problems are often not fully appreciated by others who do not have the problem which adds to the frustration of the sufferer. Memory difficulties are common among people who have dementia.

However, problems with a failing memory and simple forgetfulness are found among people with head injuries. In fact, any one of us has experienced forgetting something at one time or another.

This book follows the demand from patients, carers, researchers and referrers to health services for help with memory problems. It is intended to address some of the everyday problems that people encounter when they suffer from a poor memory, whether it is simple forgetting, a completely "blank" mind for what to do next or what they meant to say, or for more complicated and often protracted conditions such as forgetting people's names or sequences in everyday tasks.

This book is designed to guide the reader; however, for persisting problems, it is advisable to seek the opinion of the family doctor in the first instance so that a referral may be made for further specialist help.

This book details the many types of dementia and how memory problems often affect the presenting problem. It is intended to help both students and professionals understand better the conditions associated with dementia and to gain an insight into the many ways with which we can help people who have a memory difficulty.

PART I
Defining Dementia and Memory

Chapter 1

Introduction to Dementia

Background

Increasing longevity, especially of people with learning disabilities (Jancar, 1984; Wolf & Wright, 1987; Eyman et al., 1987), has brought with it a seemingly ever-increasing demand on health and social services. In particular, clinical psychology services have seen an increasing number of referrals to assess older clients who have poor cognitive functioning and to provide advice for carers about clients who have declining memory ability (Thompson, 1994a). Supportive consultation with staff and clients alike is also important, and has increased the demands on all services as the size of the older population has grown.

Identifying signs of declining memory and general cognitive functioning early on clearly has many advantages (see Huppert & Tym, 1986), including the planning and provision of specialist care for these people. Researchers and clinicians have been interested in the effects of ageing on the normal population for some considerable time (for example, Holden, 1989), and have compared common impairments, such as short-term memory (McDade & Adler, 1980), age-related memory decline (Young & Kramer, 1991), and psychophysiological differences, such as auditory event-related potentials (Muir, Squire & Blackwood, 1988). The difficulties of a differential diagnosis between depression and dementia have also been examined (Warren, Holroyd & Folstein, 1989), but the stumbling block for researchers has often been the transferability of measures to different client groups (Rosen, Mohs & Davis, 1984). Often, standardised assessments are too difficult or are culturally dependent; testing some clients results in floor or ceiling effects, and other tests are simply too demanding on a subject's attention or concentration.

Normal Ageing

In order to understand the complexities of dementia, it is worthwhile describing what happens in normal ageing, and understanding what can go wrong and gives rise to abnormal conditions such as dementia. Ageing can be distinguished in terms of biological, social and psychological factors, but there is often a great overlap and interaction between them. For example, a physical change, such as arthritis, can limit mobility, which in turn can reduce involvement in social activities or other previous sources of enjoyment (Alcott, 1993). The influence of one aspect of ageing on another should also be remembered; this is important when considering and comparing past and present cognitive functions within the same person.

Defining 'normal' is a difficult task, and it is surprising how 'normal' and 'abnormal' activities and attitudes often overlap. The blurring of boundaries occurs between different cultures, different environments or even between individuals. One misconception is to consider normality as distinct and opposite to abnormality, when in fact 'normality' refers to the 'range around the middle of a dimension (for example, height) with two extremes at opposite ends (very tall and very short), rather than one extreme' (Alcott, 1993, p. 9).

Different people have differing concepts of normality, and hence differing expectations about ageing. With the advance of medicines and technology, people generally live longer, so more people are exposed to older people and witness the variations in ageing of relatives and friends. In turn, people's understanding of normal ageing is constantly being revised, as are their expectations of themselves and others.

Normal ageing brings with it changes, not just to an individual's appearance, however subtle, but also to the higher mental functions or 'cognitive' functions. Memory can also be affected, sometimes because the individual has failed to receive information correctly, or sometimes because it can no longer be encoded or stored effectively. The effect of ageing on memory is very often one of the first of the cognitive changes to be noticed by others, and can cause considerable distress to the individual and to relatives, close friends and carers. Deterioration in memory functioning is characteristic of dementia, but it can also indicate other dysfunctions, which should always be considered in any assessment.

Generally, older people can learn as much as younger people, but more time is needed for them to achieve the same level of learning, as they cannot process and 'absorb' information as quickly as younger people. Sometimes this speed reduction becomes noticeable and marked, and leads to the onset of depression. If memory has noticeably changed, and continues to do so, it may indicate the onset of a dementing process.

Changes in language abilities can also be characteristic of dementia, but people's voice characteristics tend to change with age as part of the normal ageing process with the pitch becoming higher during the fifties, the resonance thinner, and the volume lower (Alcott, 1993). Various factors, such as smoking, stooped posture, unclean environment (for example, dust) or prolonged abuse of the voice can contribute to these changes. Ill-fitting dentures, toothlessness or weakening of the muscles involved in speech production can all hinder speech, and it is worthwhile investigating all practical aspects of a person's living environment and hygiene before drawing conclusions about a person's abilities or cognitive status.

Personality also plays a large part in normal ageing; some people adjust better than others to changes in circumstances, be it changes to their living environment, loss of occupational status, or physical changes such as decreased mobility, lack of independent transport, and so on. Some individuals become more restless or agitated at the frustration of their changed world, while others may be more placid or resigned and withdrawn. Others adapt to change, and are realistic about expectations and changes to their circumstances.

Social adaptation and sexual changes are very often major causes of people's unhappiness, yet the general expectation that older people will not be sexually active is unfounded, since there is a great deal of variation in both sexual interest and activity among all groups of people, young or older. Availability of a capable partner and acceptance of the level of a close relationship seem to be important factors in determining sexual activity or fondness. Exceptions are often found in most groupings, and some older people never cease to amaze their younger relatives with energy and wisdom sometimes absent in their younger peers!

Structural changes to the brain give rise to cognitive changes that may be noticed by others observing the individual. In normal ageing, the brain undergoes several structural changes, including a decrease in size, flattening of the surface, and increasing amounts of intracranial space (Jernigan, Zatz & Feinberg, 1980). Other microscopic and biochemical changes occur, as well as changes to the electrical activity (electrophysiological changes) within the brain (Brizzee et al., 1980; Hansch, Syndulko & Pirozzolo, 1980; Zatz, Jernigan & Ahumada, 1982a, 1982b).

Verbal skills, particularly the well-learned skills of reading, writing, vocabulary and word usage, tend to be maintained (Botwinick, 1977), and the general intellectual status of healthy older people, as measured by neuropsychological tests, tends to remain within normal limits through the eighties (Benton, Eslinger & Damasio, 1981). Arithmetical ability is also generally stable among older people (Kramer & Jarvik, 1979; Williams, 1970). Arithmetic and memory tests that show decreased performance in older people – for example, Digits Backward of the Wechsler Adult Intelligence Scale – Revised

(Wechsler, 1981a) – tend to reflect impaired concentration and mental tracking, rather than decreased cognitive functioning. However, a normal tendency for digit and letter memory span to be a little longer in the auditory than visual modality appears to increase with age (Craik, 1977; Kramer & Jarvik, 1979).

Contrary to conventional belief, normal ageing processes do not affect the immediate memory span in older people (Williams, 1970). Lezak (1983) points out that the normal intellectual decline associated with old age shows up most strikingly in four areas of intellectual activity; these can be summarised as follows:

1. The primary, or working, memory capacity of intact older people differs little from that of younger adults (Erickson, 1978), except when the amount of material to be remembered exceeds the normal primary storage capacity of six or seven items (Craik, 1977). Older people use less effective learning procedures (less elaborative encoding), and tend to show a greater differential between recall and recognition of learned material, particularly when the recognition tasks are easy (Botwinick & Storandt, 1974). Contrary to studies that indicate a progressive loss in recall of public events (Squire, 1974), Botwinick and Storandt (1980) reported that memory for remote events does not appear to change with the passage of time.

2. Diminished ability for abstract and complex conceptualisation typifies the intellectual functioning of older people (Botwinick, 1977; Denney, 1974; Reitan, 1967). The more meaningful and concrete the presentation of a reasoning problem, the greater the likelihood that people will succeed at it (Botwinick, 1978).

3. Mental inflexibility, manifesting as difficulty in adapting to new situations, solving novel problems or changing mental set, characterises intellectual performance failures of older age (Botwinick, 1978; Schaie, 1958).

4. General behavioural slowing is a predominant characteristic of ageing that affects perceptual (Kramer & Jarvik, 1979), cognitive (Botwinick, 1977; Thomas, Fozard & Waugh, 1977) and memory functions, as well as all psychomotor activity (Benton, 1977; Hicks & Birren, 1970; Welford, 1977). Accurate evaluation of older people's poor performance on any timed test must depend on careful observation and analysis of the effect of time limits on the scores, for the score alone will tell little about the effects.

Physical and Psychological Problems of Ageing

Confusion is commonly misunderstood to be a part of the dementing process, when in fact an acute confusional state is 'a consequence of change in the body's metabolism which leads to high temperature, fever and delirium, which in turn can cause temporary disorientation, memory loss, a state of "muddled perplexity", poor concentration, hallucinations, clouding of consciousness and restlessness' (Goudie, 1993, p. 29).

Unlike the situation where the person is suffering from dementia, the disorientation and confusion will improve if the underlying cause is treated. Regular check-ups are therefore important in ensuring that health problems and reactions to medication are dealt with before they lead to serious consequences. Misdiagnosis can often occur in people who are over 65 years old, mainly because certain reactions seem to indicate dementia at first glance. For example, acute confusional state can be caused by: poor diet, chest and urinary infections, heart disease, faecal impaction, sensory deprivation (for example, poor eyesight, poor hearing, social isolation), grief reaction to bereavement, and so on.

Signs such as changes in muscle tone, persistent language problems, perceptual problems and personality changes may indicate other conditions such as transient ischaemic attack (TIA) or a cerebrovascular accident ('stroke'). Haemorrhage in the blood vessels leading to the brain or in the vessels of the brain itself can result in a stroke. The cognitive changes associated with a stroke can be confused with a dementing process if the physical effects of the stroke are disguised or are subtle. Indeed, some small strokes do not cause devastating or obvious outward changes, but many small strokes that cause death to specific brain sites (multi-infarcts) often lead to dementia (Thompson & Morgan, 1996).

In Murphy's 1982 survey, about 30 per cent of people were found to be depressed. Indeed, it is the most common emotional problem affecting older adults (Goudie, 1993). Even when the condition has been properly identified, many individuals do not receive treatment with antidepressants (McDonald, 1986), or are referred for specialist therapy, such as cognitive therapy (Blackburn & Davidson, 1990). Some believe that depression in older age is 'normal', and that older people are rigid thinkers and are uncooperative. In fact, many older people adapt well to the times (for example, changes in currency, government policies, and so on) and are able to reflect on the past in order to apply their experienced skills to the present day.

Identifying the signs of dementia and depression are crucial to treatment. While it is generally not too difficult to list the signs of depression – for example, Hanley & Baikie (1984) list low mood, loss of interest, sleep disturbance, weight loss, hopelessness, helplessness, thoughts of death or suicide, preoccupation with somatic complaints, agitation, loss of energy, feelings of worthlessness and guilt, thinking and concentration disturbances and forgetfulness – it is sometimes harder to distinguish between an older person suffering from depression alone, versus depression and dementia. Some key diagnostic points for depression are also important in diagnosing dementia: forgetfulness, thinking and concentration disturbances, inability to maintain a task, and lack of concentration. Typical symptoms of depression may be compared with those of Alzheimer's-type dementia (Figure 1.1).

Normal Memory

Memory failure is a common and significant problem in dementia, hence it is important to first assess the extent to which it is a problem and for whom the problem is an obstacle.

A distinction is commonly drawn between a short-term memory system with limited capacity (a few items at most) and a storage time of seconds, and a long-term system with perhaps limitless capacity and indefinite storage time (Atkinson & Shiffrin, 1968). Short-term memory, now elaborated into the concept of 'working memory' (Baddeley, Wilson & Watts, 1995), is the system which enables a new telephone number to be remembered while dialling it – as long as there is no distraction. Long-term memory allows one to remember a familiar telephone number from day to day and year to year (Collerton, 1993). This terminology differs from commonplace use, where short-term memory is taken to be the memory for the preceding hours, days or months, and long-term memory for many years in the past.

It is now believed that there are four stages involved in memory:

1. registration;
2. encoding;
3. storage;
4. retrieval.

For information to be stored in memory, it must first be attended to, or *registered. Encoding* is the process whereby this information may be semantically or phonologically encoded (encoded in terms of meaning or sound, respectively) (Baddeley, 1978). *Storage* is the process by which information is maintained in memory. It is widely accepted that different types of knowledge appear to be stored differently, so that, for example, knowing what a person ate for lunch (episodic memory) would be stored differently from knowing the word 'lunch' means a mid-day meal (semantic memory). Cohen and Squire (1981) have subsumed these terms under 'declarative memory', and reserve a further definition, termed 'procedural memory', for skills and routines including some types of sensory memory (for example, knowing how to ride a motorbike is a *procedural* memory, knowing how the engine works is *declarative*). These functional definitions of memory have practical applications for therapists and are also more simplistic than earlier definitions. *Retrieval* is the process by which information is made available from memory, and is thought to be dependent upon a number of factors, such as the closeness of match between conditions at encoding and retrieval (Tulving, 1979), and the strategy used for retrieving memorised information (Roediger & Blaxton, 1987).

It is important for clinicians and therapists to understand the mechanisms involved in memory functioning in order to be able to recognise and treat deficits when they present as a consequence of dementia. Appreciating the complexities of memory also equips carers with extra skills to manage and support people with dementia. Scrutiny of case histories of patients examined for memory impairments has shown that people's intact memory is not always as comprehensive as one might imagine (Thompson, 1996b); indeed, people's memory functioning can be very selective (Thompson, 1995a). Selective memory is difficult to explain, but generally, people choose to remember only certain details of an event (Eich, 1984). People experiencing traumatic events sometimes repress distressing memories. The process used here is to block the retrieval of information, rather than preventing information from being memorised in the first place (Terr, 1994). Boring or over-complicated information is also selectively ignored and not retained.

Therefore, it is a constant battle for therapists and clinicians to seek out stimulating information while still achieving an objective assessment of a patient's memory functioning.

Figure 1.1   Depression and Dementia Compared

Depression	*Alzheimer-Type Dementia*
Complains of poor memory often	Unaware of memory problems often
In answer to questions requiring thought and/or concentration, says 'Don't know'	In answer to questions requiring concentration or a good memory, often confabulates and is unaware of giving wrong answer
Shows fluctuating ability and impairment on cognitive testing	Shows consistent, global impairment on cognitive testing
Poor motivation, uninterested, gives up easily	Willing to have a go
Aware of errors in any complex task, slow but successful in any complex task	Unsuccessful in tasks requiring concentration, appearing unaware of errors

Memory and Dementia

Dementia is complex; to understand its complexities, it is necessary to describe what happens in normal ageing and understanding what can go wrong and gives rise to abnormal conditions such as dementia. Ageing can be distinguished in terms of biological, social and psychological disciplines, but there is often a great overlap and interaction between them. For example, a physical change such as arthritis can limit mobility, which in turn can reduce involvement in social activities or other previous sources of enjoyment (Alcott, 1993). The influence of one aspect of ageing on another should also be remembered; this is important when considering and comparing past and present cognitive functions within the same person.

The definition of 'normal' is a difficult task and it is surprising how 'normal' and 'abnormal' activities and attitudes often overlap. The blurring of boundaries occurs between different cultures, different environments or even between individuals. A misconception is to consider normality as distinct and opposite to abnormality when in fact 'normality' refers to the 'range around the middle of a dimension (eg height) with two extremes at opposite ends (very tall and very short), rather than one extreme' (Alcott, 1993). Different people have their own opinion about normality and hence expectancies in ageing are perceived differently between individuals. With the advance of medicines and technology, people are generally living longer and

so more people are exposed to older people and are witness to
the variations in ageing of relatives and friends. In turn, people's
understanding of normal ageing is being constantly revised and so
too are their expectancies of themselves and others.

Normal ageing brings with it changes, not just to an individual's
appearances, however subtle, but also certain changes to the higher
mental functions or 'cognitive' functions (Allen, *et al.*, 1997; Freidl,
et al., 1997). Memory can also be affected (Craik, 1994; Small, *et
al*, 1995), sometimes because the individual has failed to receive
information correctly, or sometimes because it can no longer be
effectively encoded or stored (Nyberg, *et al.*, 1996). The effect of
ageing on memory, particularly episodic memory (Morris, 1994a), is
very often one of the first of the cognitive functions to be noticed
by others and can cause considerable distress to the individual
and to relatives, close friends and carers. Deterioration in memory
functioning is characteristic of dementia (Mitrushina, Uchiyama &
Satz, 1995) but it can also indicate other dysfunctions which should
always be considered in any assessment.

Memory functioning has been recognised as follows:

1. Short-term and long-term memory – Short-term memory, now
   elaborated into the concept of working memory (Baddeley, 1992),
   is the system which allows one to remember a new telephone
   number while one is dialling it, so long as one is not distracted.
   Long-term memory allows one to remember a familiar telephone
   number from day to day and year to year (Collerton, 1993).
2. Semantic and episodic memory – Different types of knowledge
   appear to be stored differently. A distinction drawn initially
   between episodic and semantic memories (Tulving, 1972) and,
   more latterly, a contrast between procedural and declarative
   memories has gained acceptance (Cohen & Squire, 1981).
   Episodic memories are for particular events, while semantic
   memories are context-free facts. For example, knowing what
   I had for breakfast is an episodic memory; knowing that the
   word 'breakfast' means a morning meal is a semantic memory
   (Collerton, 1993).
3. Declarative and procedural memory – Both semantic and
   episodic memories may be subsumed under this heading (which
   represent the memory for facts). Procedural memory is for skills
   and routines and may include some types of sensory stimuli. For
   example, knowing how to drive a car is a procedural memory,
   knowing how the engine works is declarative (Collerton, 1993).

Generally, older people can learn as much as younger people (Fisk, *et al.*, 1997), but more time is needed for them to achieve the same level of learning as they cannot process and 'absorb' information as quickly as younger people (Salthouse & Meinz, 1995). Sometimes this speed reduction becomes noticeable and marked and may accompany the onset of depression (Krishnan, 1991). If memory has noticeably changed and continues to do so it can indicate the signs of a dementing process, if it is accompanied by another failure in cognitive function (APA, 1994).

Changes in language abilities can also be characteristic of dementia, but as an effect of the normal ageing process, people's voice characteristics tend to change with age with the pitch becoming higher at the fifth decade, the resonance thinner, and the volume lower (Alcott, 1993). Various factors, such as smoking, stooped posture, unclean environment (eg dust) or prolonged abuse of the voice can contribute to these changes. Ill-fitting dentures, toothlessness or weakening of the muscles involved in speech production can all hinder speech and it is worthwhile investigating all practical aspects of a person's living environment and hygiene before drawing conclusions about a person's abilities or cognitive status.

Verbal skills, particularly the well-learned skills of reading, writing, vocabulary, and word usage, tend to be maintained (Moss & Patel, 1992); and the general intellectual status of healthy older people, as measured by neuropsychological tests, tends to remain within normal limits through the eighth decade (Simone & Baylis, 1997). Also, age-related decrement in semantic memory organisation and functioning are minimal if not absent (Goldblum, *et al.*, 1998). Arithmetic and memory tests that show decreased performance in older people, for example, Digits Backward of the Wechsler Adult Intelligence Scale - Revised (Wechsler, 1981), tend to reflect impaired concentration and mental tracking rather than decreased cognitive functioning (Parkin, Walter & Hunkin, 1995). Contrary to conventional belief, normal ageing processes do not affect the immediate memory span in older people (Nyberg, *et al.*, 1996).

Personality also plays a large part in normal ageing; some people adjust better than others to their change in circumstances, be it changes to their living environment, loss of occupational status, or physical changes such as decreased mobility, lack of independent transport, and so on. Some individuals become more restless or agitated at the frustration of their changed world whilst others may be more placid or resigned and withdrawn (Thompson, 1997). Yet others adapt to change and are realistic about expectations and changes to their circumstances. Social adaptation and sexual changes are very often major causes of people's unhappiness. However, the general expectation that older people will not be sexually active (Schiavi & Rehman, 1995) is unfounded since there is a great deal of variation in both sexual interest and activity amongst all groups of people, young or older. Availability of a capable partner and acceptance of the level of a close relationship seem to be important factors in determining sexual activity or fondness. Exceptions are often around in most groupings and some older people never cease to amaze their younger relatives with the energy and wisdom sometimes not found in their younger peers!

Structural changes to the brain give rise to cognitive changes (Daigneault & Braun, 1993; Golomb, *et al.*, 1996) that may be seen by others observing the individual. In normal ageing, the brain undergoes several structural changes including decreasing in size, flattening of the surface, and increasing amounts of intracrannial space (Aylward, *et al.*, 1997; Deb, 1997; Kesslak, *et al.*, 1994; Prasher, *et al.*, 1996). Other microscopic and biochemical changes occur as well as changes of the EEG (Holland, 2000).

Normal intellectual decline associated with old age shows up most strikingly in four areas of intellectual activity; these can be summarized as follows:

1. The primary, or working memory capacity of intact older people differs little from that of younger adults (Burack & Lachman, 1996) except when the amount of material to be remembered exceeds the normal primary storage capacity of six or seven items, as in tests of supraspan (Morris, 1996). Older people use less effective learning procedures - less elaborative encoding - and tend to show a greater differential between recall and recognition of learned material, particularly when the recognition tasks are easy (Fisk, *et al.*, 1997).
2. Diminished ability for abstract and complex conceptualization typifies the intellectual functioning of older people (Moss & Patel, 1992). The authors suggest that the more meaningful and concrete the presentation of a reasoning problem, the greater is the likelihood that people will succeed at it.
3. Mental inflexibility, appearing as difficulty in adapting to new situations, solving novel problems, or changing mental set, characterizes intellectual performance failures of older age (Moss & Patel, 1995; Sattel, *et al.*, 1993). Some authors have suggested that apparent intellectual slowness in solving problems may be due to serial versus parallel processing. Evidence for slower serial processing was found in tests of older people as compared

with younger participants (Ellis, Goldberg & Detweiler, 1996).
4. General behavioural slowing (Swearer & Kane, 1996) is a
   predominant characteristic of ageing that affects perceptual
   (Earles & Salthouse, 1995), cognitive (Sattel, *et al.*, 1993), and
   memory functions (Nyberg, *et a.*, 1996) as well as all psychomotor
   activity (Moss & Patel, 1992; Holland, 2000). Accurate evaluation
   of an older person's poor performance on any timed test must
   depend on careful observation and analysis of the effect of time
   limits on the scores, for the score alone will tell little about the
   effects of slowing per se (Lezak, 1983).

Anxiety and Dementia

Anxiety is also common and often overlooked in older people. It can
affect memory functioning and is particularly common in people with
dementia. However, it is also very common indeed in people who have
neither dementia nor problems with other cognitive functions.

Typical symptoms include: 'butterflies' in the stomach, sweating,
feelings of sickness, palpitations, and even diarrhoea. Hyperventilation
(breathing at a rate that is faster than normal) and dizziness, tightening
of the chest, and head and abdominal pains can be the result of an
acute anxiety panic attack. Some sufferers of anxiety find that their
arousal level is such that no one event or stimulus triggers their
panic attack. This is termed 'free-floating anxiety' and can be difficult
to treat, but is usually helped by practising relaxation regularly and
exploring different ways of interpreting threatening or uncomfortable
stimuli. Anxiolytic drugs can also take the edge off severe anxiety and
can help the sufferer explore new ways of coping.

There are several other conditions that might be confused with
a diagnosis of dementia in older people. Some of these include
paraphrenia (often defined as 'schizophrenia of late life'), alcohol-
related problems (such as Korsakoff's psychosis), and Parkinson's
disease, the most common, which occurs in 1 or 2 people in every
1,000 (Goudie, 1993). Figure 1.2 illustrates the similarities and
differences to dementia of several of the most common problems.

Figure 1.2   Similarities and Differences between Dementia and Other Problems

Problem	Similarities to dementia	Differences from dementia
Depression	Slow, unresponsive, poor concentration	Usually answers with accuracy though 'do not know' is frequent
Anxiety	Total failure to cope, unable to carry out daily tasks due to agitation	Insight into impaired functioning and no confabulation; when stress is minimised, ability is normal
Alcohol problems	'Immediate memory' loss, disorientation, co-ordination poor	Problems reduced when sobered up, consciousness clouded
Paraphrenia	Self-neglect, misinterprets actions/ statements	Despite some bizarre reasoning/ hallucinations, some parts of behaviour unimpaired
Parkinson's disease	Withdrawal from social activity and increase in dependency	Involvement/abilities may improve with medication
Stroke	Slowing, poor con- concentration and withdrawal, speech and language problems	Motor deficits not global with insight into loss and recovery of function possible; compensates for deficits using intact abilities

Ageism

'Ageism' has rapidly become accepted as a term, along with sexism, and refers to discrimination against people because of their age. In the next decade, it is estimated that there will be nearly 9 million people aged 65 or more. According to the Office of Population, Census and Statistics (OPCS, 1985), nearly half of these will be aged over 75 years, and more than 1 million will be at least 85 years old. Older age is something that we all face, and addressing problems such as our attitude to older people will, in turn, help us all. As Norman (1986) concludes in her paper: 'It is in our interest to combat ageism.'

Statements and descriptions of older people can make us think negatively about old age and about older people. Examples of these include the use of words relating to older age as insults (for example, 'wrinklies', 'becoming demented', 'gone doolally', and so on). Other factors, such as the lack of a high profile in society, lowers self-esteem in older people, and also makes younger people fear growing old. Associating older age with death is possibly the most negative view of growing older, and government documents on 'care for the elderly' imply that we will be overwhelmed by an older population before very long.

Attitudes towards older people have been examined in a number of ways, and it has been found that nursing and medical students become more negative in their attitudes to older people as their training progresses (Gale & Livesley, 1974). Social workers interviewed about their attitudes towards this group of people have shown that they feel that many skills needed for working with older people can be provided by unqualified social work assistants rather than qualified staff (Nicolson & Paly, 1981). Many people do not fully understand ageing and conditions related to age, such as some of the dementias, so it is perhaps understandable, though not excusable, that people generally have negative, and often incorrect, feelings and knowledge about older people.

Reversing some of these negative attitudes can be easily achieved through staff training. Recruiting staff who have a healthy respect for older people will help to promote good working practices and the correct approach; they are also more likely to pass on these skills to their work colleagues, either by instruction or by others observing them work effectively. Role plays in staff training days are increasingly used, and are usually popular with staff being trained. Providing staff with an opportunity to experience the effects of being older can also help them appreciate the needs of older people. Examples of these are: wheelchair use, wearing blindfolds or special spectacles that simulate impaired vision, wearing earplugs, using various aids, such as walking sticks and frames or specially-adapted aids such as can-openers and grippers, and so on. Part of being disabled is also having to accept adaptations to your home environment; this is sometimes met with frustration, and even anger.

Not all older people become disabled, and again, it is worthwhile reminding staff that everyone is different, and as such require different amounts and types of help. Experienced members of staff can also benefit from training, especially those who may be set in their ways; newer members of staff can likewise gain much insight into their more experienced peers' working lives through discussion and exchange of ideas during training days.

Age awareness exercises involve examining how we acquired our own prejudices (see Itzin, 1986), re-evaluating these prejudices and deciding to behave in different (and better) ways in our work settings. Increasing our own awareness and acting on these new views is infectious; hopefully, the message will then filter through to our colleagues.

Further Reading

Bayles, K.A. & Kaszniak, A. (1987), Communication and Cognition in Normal Ageing and Dementia, Philadelphia: Taylor & Francis.

Blackburn, I. & Davidson, K. (1990), Cognitive Therapy for Depression and Anxiety: A Practitioner's Guide (1st reprint), Oxford: Blackwell.

Holden, U. (1989), Neuropsychology and Ageing, London: Chapman & Hall.

Itzin, C. (1986), 'Ageism awareness training: A model for group work', in Phillipson, C., Bernard, M. & Strang, P. (eds), Dependency and Interdependency in Old Age: Theoretical Perspectives and Policy Alternatives, Beckenham: Croom Helm.

Norman, A. (1986), Aspects of Ageism: A Discussion Paper, London: Centre for Policy on Ageing.

Seligman, M.E.P. (1975), Helplessness, San Francisco: Freeman.

Stokes, G. (1995), On Being Old – The Psychology of Later Life, Brighton: Falmer Press.

Thompson, S.B.N. & Morgan, M. (1996), Occupational Therapy for Stroke Rehabilitation (2nd reprint), London: Chapman & Hall.

Wattis, J. & Church, M. (1986), Practical Psychiatry of Old Age, Beckenham: Croom Helm.

Woods, R.T. & Britton, P.G. (1985), Clinical Psychology with the Elderly, London: Croom Helm.

Chapter 2

Definition of Dementia

The definition of 'dementia' generally accepted by clinical psychologists and psychiatrists is that outlined in DSM-III-R (APA, 1987) and DSM-IV (APA, 1994). In summary, it states that for a diagnosis of dementia, there should be demonstrable evidence of impairment in short-term and long-term memory. Impairment in short-term memory (inability to learn new information) may be indicated by an inability to remember three objects after five minutes. Long-term memory impairment (inability to remember information that was known in the past) may be indicated by an inability to remember past personal information (for example, what happened yesterday, birthplace, occupation) or facts of common knowledge (for example, past prime ministers, well-known dates). The salient points of the full-length definition (all of which do not necessarily have to be present for a diagnosis of dementia are:

1. impairment of short-term and long-term memory;
2. impairment of abstract thinking;
3. impaired judgement;
4. disturbances of higher cortical function (for example, aphasia, apraxia, agnosia, constructional difficulty);
5. personality change;
6. specific organic factor;
7. absence of a non-organic factor as a reason for the symptoms (for example, major depression).

Dementia is commonly misunderstood to be a disease, when in fact it may be the result of a number of factors, and in some instances it may be reversible. Stokes and Holden (1993) have described 'primary dementia' as an extensive, organic impairment of intellect, memory and personality. It occurs in the absence of clouding of unconsciousness (without drowsiness), and is acquired, irreversible and progressive.

Among people aged over 65 years old, the prevalence (the percentage of people afflicted at a given time) of moderate to severe dementia has been estimated at between 1.3 and 6.2 per cent (Stokes & Holden, 1993). Some researchers believe that the increased life expectancy of women, coupled with the greater prevalence of dementia in people in their nineties, is the most likely reason more women than men suffer from dementia. However, most statistics come from the Western world and no prevalence studies of dementia have been documented in Third World countries.

It has been common to distinguish 'pre-senile' dementia from 'senile' dementia, both by age of onset and by type of illness. Lishman (1987) describes two types of dementia: arteriosclerotic (which may also occur as a presenile disease) and parenchymatous senile dementia. The latter, which refers to a dementing process in the parenchyma (the 'functional part' of the brain) is by far the commonest form of dementia, and is generally characterised by those deficits found in Alzheimer's disease (Ineichen, 1989; Katona, 1989; Miller & Morris, 1993). Multi-infarct dementia (Hachinski, 1983; Thompson & Morgan, 1996) is less common, and refers to the presence of small, localised areas of dead tissue in the brain produced as a result of an inadequate blood supply.

Over the years, there have been several different definitions of 'dementia', and these have varied, often according to the viewpoint of the person proposing the definition: for example, from a neuroanatomist's structural viewpoint or from a neuropsychologist's functional viewpoint. Definitions have also changed with the advent of improved technologies, such as computerised tomography (CT) scanning and magnetic resonance imaging (MRI). Dementias resulting from a stroke, for example, may be defined generally as 'multi-infarct dementia', or specifically, according to which blood vessels are involved, as in 'lacunar stroke'.

Alzheimer's Disease

Alzheimer's disease is named after a German physician, Alois Alzheimer, who first reported the disease in 1907. It is the single most common form of dementia, accounting for more than 50 per cent of cases of dementia in those over the age of 65 (Katzman, 1976). Initially, the neuropathology of Alzheimer's disease was thought to be arteriosclerotic; however, this was revised after researchers such as Corsellis and Evans (1965) and Tomlinson, Blessed and Roth (1970) consistently reported arteriosclerosis in people with a diagnosis of pre-senile dementia.

Typically, the onset is from 40 years of age onwards, with insidious degeneration until death at about two to five years following onset (Lishman, 1987; Jorm, 1990; Burns & Levy, 1994). Brain lesions in a typical Alzheimer-type patient have 'miliary', 'Fischer' or 'neuritic' plaques (Kolata, 1985), neurofibrillary tangles, and degeneration of the ends of nerve cells.

Studies of individuals in the general population with verified Alzheimer's disease, often by CT or MRI scans (for example, Shapiro, Haxby & Grady, 1992), have shown that clinical manifestations follow three stages (Schneck, Reisberg & Ferris, 1982). The first involves a subjective opinion of forgetfulness, which may be accompanied by anxiety (Mohanaruban, Sastry & Finucane, 1989). The second is characterised by severe memory loss for recent events (Inglis, 1959; Miller, 1973) with impaired delayed recall being more pronounced than impaired immediate recall (Baddeley et al., 1991). Poor concentration, impaired orientation and minimal dysphasia are also usually evidenced (Miller, 1981; Rau, 1993), with vocabulary and memory for past events remaining largely unaffected. The final stage is marked by severe disorientation, pronounced anxiety and cognitive abulia (absence or impairment of 'willpower') (Oliver & Holland, 1986).

There are also the effects of the residential setting on the elderly person (see Collacott, 1992). The level of staff support may vary according to the individual needs of the person. Identifying these factors for participants in research studies is important; however, this is not always possible, for both time and financial reasons. The impact of caring for those with dementia on staff support levels becomes more important during planning decisions and in the provision of specialist care for individuals with a learning disability who are dementing.

Each person with Alzheimer's disease will vary slightly in presentation according to personality. Emotional, behavioural and cognitive changes will also vary, but clinicians and researchers generally accept a stage model, which describes broad characteristics (Reisberg, 1983).

In the first phase, there is usually difficulty in recalling recent events, and a tendency to forget where objects have been placed.

The second recognised phase is known as the 'confusional phase'. Disorientation and word-finding difficulty is often observed.

The third phrase is characterised by a lack of purpose in the person's behaviour, which often appears bizarre.

There is still no conclusive evidence to show whether Alzheimer's disease is caused by an auto-immune disease. In one study of age-matched Alzheimer's disease sufferers and normal elderly people, significantly higher levels of brain-reactive antibodies were found in patients with Alzheimer's disease. Antibodies against central nervous system structures have been found in a number of other conditions, such as multiple sclerosis and schizophrenia (Fraser, 1988), therefore an auto-immune response may be a reaction to brain damage, rather than a primary cause of Alzheimer's disease (Curran & Wattis, 1989).

Environmental factors may have a role in triggering Alzheimer's disease in susceptible individuals. An association between Alzheimer's disease and aluminium has been formulated for several years. Neurofibrillary tangles can be induced experimentally in animals following intracerebral injection of aluminium salts (Terry & Pena, 1965), though this raises issues surrounding the transferability of results from animals (rabbits) to humans, as well as important ethical considerations. More recently, the relationship between Alzheimer's disease and aluminium in drinking water has been described (Martyn, 1989). Eighty-eight county districts in England and Wales were examined. The risk of Alzheimer's disease was found to be 1.5 times higher in districts where the mean aluminium concentration exceeded 0.11 mg/l. There have also been studies purporting the implication of certain neurotransmitters, such as acetylcholine, but so far these have been unconvincing (Curran & Wattis, 1989).

Heredity appears to have some influence on the risk of suffering from Alzheimer's disease (Breitner & Folstein, 1984; Cook, Ward & Austin, 1979; Feldman et al., 1963): close relatives of a sufferer have a greater risk of developing Alzheimer's disease (Whalley et al., 1982). The risk to relatives seems to vary depending on the age at which the disease began, and there is a decrease in risk with late onset (Stokes & Holden, 1993).

Many authorities hold the view that Alzheimer's disease and 'parenchymatous senile dementia' are identical in all respects other than age of onset (Lauter & Meyer, 1968). In the neuropathological picture, no distinguishing features, taken individually, have come to light; few neuropathologists would claim to be able to distinguish between the two with certainty on examination of the brain (Lishman, 1987). Therefore, it has been common to distinguish pre-senile Alzheimer's disease (with an onset before 65 years of age) from 'senile dementia of the Alzheimer type' (SDAT), which is generally considered to be identical, but with onset after age 65 years.

Neuropathology and Clinical Signs

Alzheimer's disease is the single most common form of dementia, accounting for between 1% and 4% of the population per year, rising by half decade from its lowest level at ages 65 to 7o years to rates that approach 4% over the age of 85 years (DeKosky, 2001).

Initially, the neuropathology of Alzheimer's disease was thought to be arteriosclerotic; however, this was revised after researchers such as Corsellis and Evans (1965) and Tomlinson, Blessed and Roth (1970) consistently reported no arteriosclerosis in people with a late onset Alzheimer's disease.

The clinical diagnosis of Alzheimer's disease is said to be correct 75% to 90% of the time (Morris, 1999). According to Dickson (2001), accuracy is highest for neurologists specialising in memory disorders and lowest for general practitioners, who have a tendency to overdiagnose Alzheimer's disease. The clinical accuracy also tends to be lower for older patients who often have mixed pathology rather than a single cause of dementia (Mendez, *et al.*, 1992). The only clinical means of establishing a definite diagnosis is by microscopic examination of brain tissue as there are no laboratory tests and neither sophisticated imaging techniques nor detailed neuopsychological evaluation can specify Alzheimer's disease categorically (Dickson, 1999).

Typically, the onset is from 40 years of age onwards with insidious degeneration until death at about six years following onset (Lishman, 1987; Jorm, 1990; Burns & Levy, 1994). The brain invariably displays a degree of atrophy; however, age-associated atrophy and the normal variability in brain size preclude a diagnosis based solely on gross examination of the brain (Dickson, 2001). Atrophy of the medial portion of the temporal lobe is often disproportionate to other areas of the cortex. In most cases, the primary sensory and motor cortices are relatively spared and on sectioning the brain, the lateral ventricles are usually dilated and the hippocampus and amygdala are atrophic (Dickson, 2001). More specific neuronal alterations accompany neuronal and synaptic loss. The most important of these alterations is paired helical filaments which are intraneuronal proteinaceous structures that are composed by an abnormal form of tau protein (see Cooper, *et al.*, 1995; Dickson, 1997; 1998; 2001; Dickson, *et al.*, 1995).

Studies of individuals in the general population with Alzheimer's disease, verified by neuropathology, have shown the clinical manifestations to follow three stages (Schneck, Reisberg & Ferris, 1982). The first involves a subjective opinion of forgetfulness which may be accompanied by anxiety (Mohanaruban, Sastry & Finucane, 1989). The second is characterized by severe memory loss for recent events (Reisberg, 1983) with an impaired delayed recall being more pronounced than for immediate recall (Baddeley, *et al.*, 1991). Poor concentration, impaired orientation and minimal dysphasia are also usually evidenced (Rau, 1993), with vocabulary and memory for past events remaining largely unaffected. The final stage is marked by severe disorientation and cognitive abulia, ie absence or impairment of 'willpower' (Oliver, 1999; Oliver & Holland, 1986). Anxiety and other affective disorders are declining in the final stage (Reisberg, 1983).

There are also the effects of the residential setting on the elderly person (see Collacott, 1992). The level of staff support may vary according to the individual needs of the person. These factors become more important during planning decisions and in the provision of specialist care for individuals with a learning disability who are dementing.

Each person with Alzheimer's disease will vary slightly in presentation according to personality. Emotional, behavioural and cognitive changes will also vary, but generally accepted by clinicians and researchers is a stage model which describes broad characteristics (Reisberg, 1983).

In the first phase, the 'forgetfulness phase', there is usually difficulty in recalling recent events, and a tendency to forget where objects have been placed (Greene, Hodges & Baddeley, 1995). Names of people and places, previously familiar, may be poorly recalled and a general disorientation persists and poor short-term memory (Goldblum, *et al.*, 1998). Abstract thinking, inability to concentrate on tasks and a marked lack of curiosity are also typical presentations and there may also be emotional changes such as anxiety and irritability and the 'new' or unexpected will be feared or disliked (Goudie, 1993; Thompson, 1997). Denial is also sometimes seen in presentation of people with Alzheimer's disease (Thompson, 1997).

Some researchers warn of the importance of accounting for attentional components in studies examining memory in Alzheimer's disease; this is because memory and attention are interrelated cognitive processes that are most likely to influence the functioning of each other and yet they are difficult to distinguish in psychological experiments (Simone & Baylis, 1997).

The second recognised phase is known as the 'confusional phase'. Increasingly poor attention span and a decline in generalised intellectual performance is seen with a deteriorating memory. Disorientation in place, word-finding difficulty and other changes to speech may be seen (Goldblum, *et al.*, 1998). Complex tasks are performed with difficulty, sometimes in a clumsy or inaccurate manner and often the skills the person learned last will be lost first. Hence the skills necessary for social independence and vocational skills are usually the first skills to be reduced or lost completely. Together with failing memory comes the concealment of these deficits by rationalising or confabulating events (ie providing an imaginary account of events or actions). Lack of interest in news and surroundings follows relatively quickly and can be extremely distressing to family and friends (Thompson, 1997).

The third phase, the 'dementia phase', is characterized by a lack of purpose in the person's behaviour which appears disjointed and sometimes bizarre. Remaining intellectual and self-care abilities require constant supervision as people in this phase undergo further deterioration in memory capacity, calculating ability (dyscalculia) and aspects of language are severely affected and eventually lost. Constant assistance is required for self-care skills such as grooming, dressing, toileting and for feeding. A progressive physical wasting can also be seen which will mean help with walking. Sometimes one or two years of life will follow in an almost vegetative state until death.

Environmental factors may have a role in triggering Alzheimer's disease in susceptible individuals. An association between Alzheimer's disease and aluminium has been formulated for several years (eg McDowell, 2001). However, there is more compelling contradictory evidence (eg Flaten, 2001). There have also been studies in the past purporting the implication of cholinergic neurotransmitters, such as acetylcholine, but these have been unconvincing (Curran & Wattis, 1989). Other risk factors, associated with Alzheimer's disease, have also been reported, for example, diabetes mellitus (Luchsinger, *et al.*, 2001).

Heredity appears to be of some importance to the risk of suffering from Alzheimer's disease. The identification of gene mutations and polymorphisms that either cause Alzheimer's disease or significantly increase the risk for developing it have enabled the creation of realistic rodent models of the disease (Chapman, *et al.*, 2001). However, whilst animals expressing mutated human amyloid precursor protein and presenilin-1 show dramatic parallels to Alzheimer's disease, as yet, none of the models appear to capture the full range of pathologies that characterise the human disease (Chapman, *et al.*, 2001).

The idea that genes can influence behavioural predispositions is becoming increasingly tractable (eg Isles & Wilkinson, 2000). In imprinted genes one allele is silenced according to its parental origin resulting in the inheritance of traits down the maternal or paternal line, in contrast to the more frequent mode of inheritance to the parental origin of the allele (Isles & Wilkinson, 2000). Hence, it has been suggested that genes may play an important determinant of behavioural outcome which might impact on such diseases as Alzheimer's disease.

As sporadic Alzheimer's disease is on the increase (Engelborghs & De Deyn, 2001) with growing demands on our medical services (DeKosky, 2001), there is a increasing need for early diagnosis. Cerebrospinal fluid (CSF) levels of protein tau have been shown to be significantly increased in patients with Alzheimer's disease (Andreasen, *et al.*, 1998; Andreasen, *et al.*, 1999; Hulstaert, *et al.*,

1999). In recent years, it has become apparent that the amyloid component of senile plaques may be the key molecule in the pathology of Alzheimer's disease (Bayer, *et al.*, 2001). Also, evidence has shown that an allele 4 of apolipoprotein E (ApoE) is a genetic risk factor for Alzheimer's disease underlining the possible role of ApoE in the physiopathology of Alzheimer's disease (Hofman, *et al.*, 1997; Mahley & Rall, 2000; Merched, *et al.*, 1997).

By measuring CSF ApoE level, findings show that an increased level corresponds with an increase of mRNA ApoE in the brains of Alzheimer's disease patients (Merched, *et al.*, 1997; Nemes, *et al.*, 2001). Hence, Merched and colleagues (1997) concludes that CSF ApoE level seems to be a reflection of neuronal damage and/or an inflammatory reaction that may be common to Alzheimer's disease and other neurological and related diseases.

It would seem, therefore, that close relatives of a sufferer do have a greater risk of developing Alzheimer's disease (Myers & Goate, 2001). However, only a small per centage is due to gene mutations and apolipoprotein E4 is responsible for some 17 % of these cases (Fullerton, *et al.*, 2000; Saunders, 2000; Wang, *et al.*, 2000). The risk to relatives seems to vary depending on the age at which the disease began; and there is a decrease in risk with late age onset (Stokes & Holden, 1993). Further prognostic studies are needed (eg Ruitenberg, *et al.*, 2001).

Neuropsychology

In normal functioning, several types of information may be processed at once, possibly from a variety of sources. An example of this might be holding a conversation or driving a car. These types of activities break down relatively rapidly in patients with dementia, even at the early stages. Alberoni, *et al.* (1992) reported that Alzheimer-type patients are particularly handicapped in keeping track of conversations involving several people. They also often have problems in remembering who said 'what' and 'when' (Thompson, 1997).

(i) Selective attention A specific component of executive processes (Baddeley, 1998), is selective attention (Morris, 1996). This has been most extensively investigated in relation to attentional shifts in spatial tasks (Simone & Baylis, 1997). Some researchers have distinguished between the three components that underlie attentional shifting, namely, engaging or focusing, shifting, and disengagement of attention (Morris, 1996).

In the auditory domain, deficits in selective attention may be measured by the dichotic listening task (Mohr, et al., 1990). Visual selective attention deficits may be evaluated by using visual display units to present stimuli via a screen (Filoteo, et al., 1992). There is substantial evidence that shifting of attention is controlled, in part, by the posterior parietal region of the brain (LaBerge, 1990). Because of the substantial functional impairment in the posterior parietal cortex in Alzheimer's disease, a specific attentional deficit would be predicted and indeed, has been found to be the case (Parasuraman, et al., 1992).

However, more recently, researchers have found that whilst patients with Alzheimer's disease have deterioration in both memory and attention, the progression of Alzheimer's disease is more closely related to deterioration of spatial memory (Simone & Baylis, 1997). The authors suggest that memory and attention are interrelated cognitive processes but are often difficult to distinguish in patient participant experiments.

(ii) Sustained attention In the early stages of Alzheimer's disease, the patient is essentially 'alert' and able to take in information to a certain level of efficiency. At a clinical level, 'alertness' readily translates into the cognitive concept of vigilance, the ability to detect a stimulus and respond readily (Morris, 1996). This is typically assessed using tasks in which a target occurs infrequently and unpredictably and has to be discriminated from other unpredictable items (Parasuraman & Giambra, 1991).

Interestingly, Alzheimer' disease patients were found to be no worse than controls on a tone discrimination task (Lines, *et al.*, 1991), but if the task complexity is increased, their vigilance becomes worse (Berardi, *et al.*, 1992). However, as a discrimination between non-Alzheimer's disease patients, such tasks do not appear to be of particular help clinically (Morris, 1996).

(iii) Working Memory Model Information processing, attention and memory are successfully characterised by the Working Memory Model developed by Alan Baddeley and colleagues (Baddeley, 1986; 1992; 1996; Baddeley & Hitch, 1974). The model proposes a Central Executive System (CES) which functions to co-ordinate and schedule mental operations including the processing and immediate storage of information. This incorporates the notion of a 'scratch pad' system which holds and manipulates information simultaneously.

The CES has limited resources, hence the decline in performance associated with trying to combine two attentionally demanding mental operations. A cluster of peripheral systems support the functioning of the CES. This includes a specialised Articulatory Loop System (ALS), responsible for recycling verbally encodable information, such as when a person tries to keep in mind a telephone number for a short period or understand a grammatically complicated sentence.

In the visuospatial domain, there is the visuospatial scratchpad (VSSP) which maintains visuospatial imagery. These components of the model are interacting continuously with the CES devoting varying degrees of processing resources to each component depending on the task (Fig 2.1). This is not the only model explaining sequencing and executive phenomena (eg Shallice, 1988; Furster, 1993), but it has provided a useful framework for studying cognitive impairment in dementia which has in part been characterised as a dysexecutive syndrome (Morris, 1986; Baddeley, *et al.*, 1986; Becker, 1988).

Figure 2.1   Schematic based on Baddeley's (1992) Working Memory Model

THE CENTRAL EXECUTIVE SYSTEM

^   ^

^   ^

^   ^

VISUOSPATIAL   ARTICULATORY

SKETCHPAD   LOOP SYSTEM

^   ^

^   ^

^   ^

THE CENTRAL EXECUTIVE SYSTEM

The peripheral systems of the Working Memory Model (Baddeley, 1992; 1998) are co-ordinated by the CES. The most extensively studied is the ALS which recycles verbal material in a relatively automatic fashion. For example, when remembering a string of digits, as in the digit span test of the Wechsler Adult Intelligence Scale Revised (Wechsler, 1981), the material is cycled continuously through the ALS to keep it in memory. A series of studies indicate that this system is unimpaired in Alzheimer's disease (Morris, 1984; 1987a,b; 1992). The evidence comes from experiments where patients are required to recall short lists of digits or words but the functioning of the ALS is suppressed by requiring them to mouth an irrelevant word (such as the word 'the'), effectively blocking articulatory rehearsal. 'Articulatory suppression' of this sort was found to have quantitatively the same effect on digits or words recall in Alzheimer's disease patients as in normal subjects. Thus, the equivalent loss of function without articulatory rehearsal shows the potency of the system to recycle verbal material is undiminished in Alzheimer's disease (Morris, 1992).

The visual counterpart of the ALS is the visuospatial sketchpad which functions to retain visuospatial memory in immediate memory (Baddeley, 1992; 1998). For example, if a person's attention is diverted momentarily from a visual scene, they will still maintain the memory of that scene for a short period. This ability helps the person maintain a sense of visual continuity when, for example, moving around the room.

Although this ability has not been investigated extensively, there is evidence for significant impairment in visuospatial memory in Alzheimer's disease (Morris, 1994a). Firstly, patients with Alzheimer's disease have difficulty in a visual analogue of verbal span - the patient observes the experimenter tapping out a sequence on an array of nine blocks (or printed coloured squares as in the Wechsler Memory Scale Revised - Wechsler, 1988) in front of them and then has to immediately repeat the sequence of taps from memory. This block span performance has been found to be impaired consistently (Spinnler, *et al*, 1988).

Secondly, there is a measure known as the 'delayed matching to sample task' where an item is shown to the patient followed by a short delay followed by the same item with another or several others. The patient is required to pick out the item seen before. By varying the delay it is possible to see how fast memory for the item decays. Sahakian, *et al.* (1988) used a version in which a pattern was shown on a computer screen and the patient had to identify the pattern from four others. Early Alzheimer's disease patients were found to show more rapid forgetting than normal older controls. A later study by Money, *et al.* (1992) found a similar impairment using filled circles of different sizes, but Alzheimer's disease patients were impaired when there was no delay between presentation and choice and showed the same rate of forgetting as the controls. Both studies, therefore, showed a substantial impairment in the performances of Alzheimer's disease patients.

Baddeley, *et al.* (1991) favours a localisationalist view; impairment in Alzheimer-type patients may be explained in terms of the dysexecutive syndrome and frontal lobe dysfunction. This links the notion of the CES to the Norman and Shallice (1986) model of attentional control which assumes that most ongoing actions are controlled by establishing routines. The routines or 'schemas' are mutually inhibitory and can be triggered by environmental events. Where they are insufficient to generate appropriate activity, a higher-level system, the Supervisory Attentional System (SAS) comes into play which is involved in coping with novel circumstances or problem-solving activity (Morris, 1994b).

Shallice (1988) relates an impairment in the SAS to the difficulties patients with frontal lobe damage have in problem-solving. The conceptual link between the CES and the SAS has been introduced by Baddeley, *et al.* (1991), who suggests that an SAS impairment also results in the reduced capacity to direct and control attentional resources. Thus an impairment in the SAS may be closely analogous to the dysexecutive syndrome seen in Alzheimer's disease. Indeed, Alzheimer's disease patients do have damage to their frontal lobes (Morris, 1994b).

Vascular Dementia

Vascular dementia, previously known as 'Multi-infarct dementia' is a fluctuating and remitting vascular-type dementia which is characterised by an abrupt onset (Stokes & Holden, 1993). It is defined as an arteriosclerotic dementia, and may occur in the mid-forties, but is usually seen in people in their seventies and eighties. Vascular dementia is the second most common form of dementia, after Alzheimer's disease. The aetiology of this type of dementia is a series of small strokes, which may vary between individuals in frequency, intensity and also in location in the brain. Loss of specific cognitive functioning, minor neurological signs (such as weakness in the muscles on one side of the body, or slurring of speech) and sometimes periods of confusion may occur. Physical disability is usually not severe, unlike that following a severe stroke. Following the infarct, there is usually limited improvement until the next episode, which can take place after a few weeks, months or even up to a year later. The deterioration in cognitive functioning and mild disability is usually a step-wise process, compared with Alzheimer's disease, which is often an insidious, gradual deterioration in functioning. Many people suffering from vascular dementia do not reach the end stage, and die from a major stroke. However, early recognition and treatment of the underlying disease (such as hypertension, arteriosclerosis or cardiac disease) may inhibit further deterioration.

The clinical diagnosis of vascular dementia is similar to that of Alzheimer's disease. Extensive diagnostic studies are completed to rule out reversible aetiologies, but if there is a history of one or more strokes or transient ischaemic attacks, a diagnosis of vascular dementia is more likely, but not definite (Brust, 1983). Hachinski's Ischaemic Score may help to differentiate between Alzheimer's disease and vascular dementia (Hachinski et al., 1975; Rosen, Terry & Fuld, 1980). Alzheimer's disease and vascular dementia may, of course, coexist in the same patient.

Neuropsychology

Vascular dementia is a fluctuating and remitting vascular type dementia which is characterized by an abrupt onset (Stokes & Holden, 1993; Markesberry, 1998; Skoog, Kalaria & Breteler, 1999). The diagnosis demands neuropathology not showing Alzheimer's disease changes and is defined in DSM-IV as follows:

A. The development of multiple cognitive deficits manifested by both

1) memory impairment (impaired ability to learn new information or to recall previously learned information)

(2) one (or more) of the following cognitive disturbances:

(a) aphasia (language disturbance)
(b) apraxia (impaired ability to carry out motor activities despite intact motor function)
(c) agnosia (failure to recognize or identify objects despite intact sensory function)
(d) disturbance in executive functioning (ie planning, organizing, sequencing, abstracting).

B. The cognitive deficits in Criteria A1 and A2 each cause significant impairment in social or occupational functioning and represent a significant decline from a previous level of functioning.

C. Focal neurological signs and symptoms (eg exaggeration of deep tendon reflexes, extensor plantar response, pseudobulbar palsy, gait abnormalities, weakness of an extremity) or laboratory evidence indicative of cerebrovascular disease (eg multiple infarctions involving cortex and underlying white matter) that are judged to be etiologically related to the disturbance.

D. The deficits do not occur exclusively during the course of a delirium. (p 146).

Vascular dementia is the second most common form of dementia, after Alzheimer's disease (Skoo, Kalaria & Breteler, 1999). The aetiology, or cause of this type of dementia is a series of small strokes which may vary between individuals in frequency, intensity and also in location in the brain (de Groot, *et al.*, 2000a,b; Thompson & Morgan, 1996). Loss of specific cognitive functioning, (eg immediate memory functioning deficits, loss of visuospatial ability, attention and concentration deficits), minor neurological signs (such as weakness in the muscles on one side of the body, or slurring of speech) and sometimes periods of confusion may occur (Thompson, 1999a). Physical disability is usually not severe unlike that following a severe stroke. Following the infarct, there is usually limited improvement until the next episode which can take place after a few weeks, months or even up to a year later (Thompson, 1999a).

The deterioration in cognitive functioning and mild disability is usually a step-wise process, as compared with Alzheimer's disease which is often an insidious gradual deterioration in functioning (Thompson, 1999a). However, recent studies have indicated that there may be a vascular connection with Alzheimer's disease (O'Brien, *et al.*, 1996; Rhodin & Thomas, 2001) in that cerebral vascular changes in patients with Alzheimer's disease probably precede the neuronal damage and dementia. Many people suffering from vascular dementia do not reach the end stage and die from a major stroke. However, early recognition and treatment of the underlying disease, such as hypertension, arteriosclerosis, or cardiac disease may inhibit further deterioration (Thompson, 1999a; Thompson & Morgan, 1996).

Researchers have attempted to devise methods for discriminating between Alzheimer's disease and vascular dementia such as CSF investigation (eg Nemes, *et al.*, 2001). However, determination of $N^\varepsilon(\gamma$-glutamyl) lysine concentration in CSF have so far not provided the discrimination available at post-mortem (Nemes, *et al.*, 2001). The clinical diagnosis of vascular dementia is similar to that of Alzheimer's disease; indeed, they share the common risk factor, apolipoprotein E4 (Dickson, 2001).

In terms of cognitive functioning, patients diagnosed with subcortical ischaemic vascular dementia tested on recognition memory and verbal fluency performed better than Alzheimer's disease patients on the recognition memory tests (Tierney, *et al.*, 2001). Criteria for the diagnosis for ischaemic vascular dementia (IVD) has been made more rigorous by some groups of researchers (eg Chui, *et al.*, 1992; Román, *et al.*, 1993). Chui and colleagues (1992), for example, have drawn up a new set of criteria that describe 'probable IVD', 'possible IVD', 'definite IVD', or 'mixed dementia' (see Chui, *et al.*, 1992). Román and colleagues (1993), on the other hand, suggest that better interobserver agreement in the diagnosis of dementia was achieved from using the World Health Organisation International Classification of Diseases (ICD-10NA) (WHO, 1992). Diagnosis of dementia requires the presence of a 'decline in memory and intellectual abilities that causes impaired functioning in daily living' (Román, *et al.*, 1993).

'Impaired functioning in daily living' was accepted as a criterion for epidemiologic studies of vascular dementia because it would ensure that the changes are more than incidental and would increase specificity (Román, et al., 1993). Chui and colleagues (1992) also included 'interference with the conduct of the patient's customary affairs of life' as a requirement for the diagnosis of ischaemic vascular dementia. The impairment should be due to cognitive deficits and not to physical handicaps produced by stroke.

For the diagnosis of vascular dementia, Román and colleagues (1993) have suggested that cognitive decline should be demonstrated by loss of memory and deficits in at least two other domains, including orientation, attention, language-verbal skills, visuospatial abilities, calculations, executive functions, motor control, abstraction, and judgement. For diagnosis, memory deficits may not be as severe as in Alzheimer's disease, but single or isolated defects in cognition such as amnesic states, aphasias, and apraxias, do not meet the requirements. Therefore, although single cognitive deficits do not qualify,

> single lesions may produce vascular dementia when causing alteration of memory and at least two other cognitive functions of sufficient severity to cause impairment in daily living (Román *et al.*, 1993, p 253).

Using the Mini-Mental State Examination (MMSE) (Folstein, Folstein & McHugh, 1975), Tatemichi and colleagues (1991) have found 84% sensitivity, 76% specificity, a false-positive rate of 46%, and a false-negative rate of 6%, supporting the use of the MMSE for screening dementia stroke patients when adjustments are made to account for false positives. Other tests that could be useful for vascular dementia include the four-word memory test with 10-minute delayed recall, the cube-drawing test for copy, a verbal fluency test, Luria's alternating hand sequence or finger rings, the letter cancellation test for neglect, the reaction-time test, and the grooved pegboard test (Cummings, 1992; Grafman, 1991). The Mattis Dementia Rating Scale (Paul, *et al.*, 2001) has also been recognised as serving as a useful diagnostic tool in this respect.

To be considered as evidence in favour of vascular dementia, the radiological findings should fulfil minimum standards for both severity and topography (Román, *et al.*, 1993). In contrast, the California criteria (Chui, *et al.*, 1992), require 'two or more ischaemic strokes with at least one infarct outside the cerebellum'. Criteria from the National Institute of Neurological Disorders (NINDS) with support from the Association Internationale pour la Recherche et l'Enseignement en Neurosciences (AIREN) (Román, *et al.*, 1993), recognise that a single lesion may cause vascular dementia and accept radiological lesions regardless of location as evidence of cerebrovascular disease. This picture is further complicated when considering a differential diagnosis (Dickson, 2001; Krishnan & McDonald, 1995; Rao, 1998).

Subcortical Arteriosclerotic Encephalopathy

A rare variant of arteriosclerotic dementia was first described by Binswanger (1894) under the term 'encephalitis subcorticalis chronica progressiva' (known later as Binswanger's disease). It has come into greater prominence as a result of certain distinctive findings on CT scans, and the realisation that diffuse white matter damage is probably more common than previously suspected in patients with dementia (Lishman, 1987). The cognitive failure in such patients seems to be attributable to the pronounced white matter changes since the cerebral cortex is often only mildly affected, if at all.

Associated clinical features are of a slowly-evolving dementia, associated with focal neurological deficits, usually in hypertensive patients in their fifties and sixties. Caplan and Schoene (1978) have clarified the picture from their cases known before post-mortem. They noted persistent hypertension, a history of acute strokes, a lengthy course, and dementia accompanied by prominent motor signs, and usually by pseudobulbar palsy. The distinctive clinical manifestation, however, was the subacute progression of focal neurological deficits. Such deficits commonly developed in a gradual fashion over some weeks or months, the picture then stabilising, with long plateau periods lasting for months, or occasionally years. This feature appeared to separate the Binswanger patients from those whose dementia rested on large vessel occlusions or on a lacunar state without accompanying white matter demyelination.

Pick's Disease

This is much less common than Alzheimer's disease, yet it was first described earlier, in 1892. The aetiology is uncertain, but there is evidence to suggest a genetic component. Most often, this dementia is seen between the ages of 45 and 60, though some researchers (for example, Lishman, 1987) suggest onset peaks between 50 and 60 years, with onset possible from the twenties onwards. Lishman also suggests that the course is slower than with Alzheimer's disease, with death following in two to ten years. Clinically, it is often suggested that frontal lobe-type changes are the earliest signs, hence diminished drive, tactless and grossly insensitive behaviour, a fatuous and vacant expression, and disinhibition are suggested as early signs rather than impairment of memory. Some researchers feel that there is no difference in the prognosis compared to Alzheimer's disease, especially since impairment of intellect does eventually follow and memory capacity and functioning is also not spared. Often perseverative speech (stereotyped repetition of words and phrases) is said to be characteristic, but again, there is disagreement among researchers and clinicians.

Pathologically, there is a degree of generalised atrophy, combined with particular shrinkage of the frontal and temporal lobes. Senile plaques, neurofibrillary tangles and vascular changes are generally absent, but there is usually considerable loss of myelin in the white matter of affected lobes. Despite the fact that clinical and pathological features differ from those of Alzheimer's disease, Lishman (1983) concedes that a realistic or truly accurate diagnosis usually has to wait until post-mortem.

Confusion over diagnosis has given rise to a number of reports (for example, Cummings & Duchen, 1981; Klüver & Bucy, 1939) including a discussion and comparison with Klüver-Bucy syndrome (Bucy & Klüver, 1955). This syndrome was originally produced in monkeys by ablating both temporal lobes, including the amygdalae, unci, and hippocampi regions of the brain. The resulting behavioural syndrome consisted of prominent oral tendencies, emotional blunting, altered dietary habits, hypermetamorphosis (tendency to react by exploring environmental stimuli as soon as they are noticed), sensory agnosia-like behaviour involving both vision and hearing, and hypersexuality (Cummings & Duchen, 1981). Similar behavioural changes have been observed in those previously diagnosed with Pick's disease.

Parkinson's Disease

This neurological condition affects the basal ganglia, an area in the subcortical part of the brain responsible for co-ordinating motor action. Tremor, rigidity, slowness of movement and postural problems are all symptoms that can occur. The most common form of the disease is idiopathic (unexplained) Parkinson's disease which occurs in 1 or 2 people in every 1,000 (Goudie, 1993). About two-thirds of sufferers of Parkinson's disease show the first signs between 50 and 69 years of age. Similar symptoms can also occur as a side-effect of some forms of medication, such as the neuroleptic drugs used for treating psychotic illnesses like schizophrenia.

A proportion of end-stage Parkinson's disease patients also suffer from dementia. Some researchers consider that this type of dementia is consistent with the presentation of Alzheimer's disease (Knight, Godfrey & Shelton, 1988), while others believe that it is primarily a subcortical dementia (Cummings, 1986). In the early stages of Parkinson's disease, cognitive functioning is usually intact. However, due to the severe motor difficulties which occur, and the fact that about two-fifths of Parkinson's patients have been found to suffer from depression related to difficulties in adjusting to the illness (or to chemical imbalance caused by the disease, which increases the person's susceptibility to depression), the condition is sometimes misinterpreted as dementia (Baldwin & Byrne, 1989; Goudie, 1993).

Commonly, treatment of Parkinsonian symptoms includes medication, usually laevodopa (L-dopa). This slows down but does not completely halt the progress of the disease. The drug itself, taken over a period of time, can cause side-effects which include hallucinations and disinhibited behaviour. Careful monitoring of medication is important. Alternative and more radical approaches have included surgical excision of the globus pallidus, but this is not yet routinely carried out, although, so far, it has shown some promising results.

There is often a role for speech and language therapists, occupational therapists and physiotherapists, as well as clinical psychologists. The latter can provide useful advice and support to help the sufferer and their family adjust to the changes the disease brings with it, which often involves treating depression in the patient.

Huntington's Disease

Huntington's disease, sometimes also known as 'Huntington's chorea' (Huntington, 1872) is a rare disease characterised by choreiform movements combined with dementia, hence 'chorea'. Since Huntington's original account in 1872, cases have been reported from all over the world, and no race appears to be immune. Prevalence varies markedly between studies; very high figures have been reported from Tasmania, while in Japan the disease appears to be extremely rare. Myrianthopoulos (1966) has estimated the overall prevalence to be 4–7 cases in 100,000. In the United Kingdom, surveys have indicated 5.2 cases per 100,000 for the West of Scotland (Bolt, 1970), and 6.3 cases per 100,000 in Northamptonshire, where detailed lineages havebeen kept for many years (Oliver, 1970). In one part of Scotland, the Moray Firth, a remarkably dense focus has been reported, with the equivalent of 560 cases per 100,000 in a small fishing community on the east coast of Ross-shire (Lyon, 1962).

The disease is associated with a single, autosomal, dominant gene with virtually a 100 per cent rate of manifestation (Lishman, 1987). Approximately half of the offspring of an affected person can therefore be expected to develop the disorder, with equal incidence in males and females. Cases in Massachusetts and Connecticut have been traced back to emigrants from England, principally to three men and their wives who left from Bures in Suffolk in 1630, and thereafter produced 11 generations of children with the disease (Vessie, 1932).

The onset of the disease is usually between the ages of 25 and 50, with an average in the mid-forties (Lishman, 1987). Variation is wide, and onset has been reported in childhood and in extreme old age. There is evidence that the disease follows a more severe course when onset is early rather than late, and that emotional disturbance is more prominent as a premonitory feature. Most researchers agree that psychiatric changes are often present for some considerable time before chorea or intellectual impairment develops. A change in personality may be marked, the patient may become morose and quarrelsome, or slowed, apathetic and neglectful of themselves or of their home. Paranoid developments may be the earliest change, with marked sensitivity and ideas of reference.

The typical early choreic movements consist of commonly-distributed and irregularly-timed muscle jerks, brief in duration and unpredictable in their appearance. With worsening of the disease, the pathological nature of the disturbance becomes more obvious. The movements are abrupt, jerky, rapid and repetitive, but vary from one muscle group to another. One half of the body may be massively affected in 'hemichorea', and involvement of the diaphragm and bulbar muscles may lead to jerky breathing, explosive, staccato speech, dysphagia, and difficulty in protruding the tongue (Lishman, 1987).

The dementia seen with Huntington's chorea is commonly very insidious in development. General inefficiency in the management of daily affairs is usually the presenting feature, rather than failing memory. As Lishman (1987) reports, this relative sparing of memory as the disease progresses is consonant with the pathological finding that the limbic areas of the brain are often less affected than in other dementias. The special features of the dementia in Huntington's chorea seem to be poor cognitive ability generally, but a lack of language disorder or other focal cortical deficits, suggesting that much of the origin of the disease lies in the subcortical areas, rather than in the cortex. The course, after the first definite presentations of the disease, is much longer than other dementias, but with a wide variation between 13 to 16 years, or more slowly over several decades.

Genetic counselling is the only current method of curtailing the disease, and is indicated on humanitarian and economic grounds. In Barette and Marsden's (1979) survey, most relatives stated that they preferred to know the painful facts as soon as possible, and the majority were then prepared to restrict their families or have no children whatever.

Creutzfeldt-Jakob Disease

Creutzfeldt-Jakob disease (CJD) is a rare disease, with about 20 new cases estimated in the United Kingdom each year (Lishman, 1987). However, early indications suggest this figure may be rising. It was first described by Creutzfeldt (1920) and Jakob (1921). The disorder consists of a dementing illness which runs a rapid course, usually accompanied by a number of prominent neurological symptoms. Florid psychiatric symptoms, such as delusions or hallucinations are often seen, but many different clinical pictures of the disorder have been reported, making diagnosis difficult. The neurological changes typically include an accent on structures additional to the cerebral cortex itself: the subcortical nuclear masses, cerebellum and brain stem and cord.

The disease usually arises sporadically, though review of a large case corpus world-wide has shown that a positive family history is obtained in about 15 per cent of cases (Masters et al., 1970). Investigations have been carried out into various transmissible agents and have focused on similarities between kuru and CJD (Gibbs et al., 1968), kuru being transmissible to chimpanzees by brain innoculation.

The precise nature of the transmissible agent involved in CJD remains elusive, however. It belongs to the category of 'unconventional' or 'slow' viruses involved in other central nervous system disorders, including CJD and kuru in man, scrapie in sheep and goats, and transmissible mink encephalopathy (Lishman, 1987). Although several definite geographical clusters of cases have been reported in people unrelated genetically to one another, no conclusive cause has been confirmed. From such epidemiological surveys, it has been possible to conclude that incubation periods of CJD often last for many years. The possibility remains that while intimate exposure to other sufferers of the disease is insufficient to cause the disease, it may contribute in persons who have inherited special genetic susceptibility.

The possibility of contracting the disease through eating animal products has been raised by analogy with scrapie in sheep (Roos,

1981). Firm evidence had not been forthcoming until more recently, yet concern arose at Kahana et al.'s (1974) discovery of a very high incidence of CJD among Libyan Jewish immigrants to Israel, thought possibly to be related to the eating of sheep's eyeballs, but significant familial clusterings were ultimately shown to account for the excess (Alter, Neugut & Kahana, 1978; Neugut et al., 1979).

The public consumption of British beef came under scrutiny in 1996, with widespread media coverage warning against beefburgers and other products containing bovine specified offal that may carry the variant in 'mad cows', bovine spongiform encephalopathy (BSE). Research is continuing and is spearheaded by the CJD Surveillance Unit in Edinburgh, Scotland. However, despite a growing number of reported teenage sufferers of CJD and comparative neuropathological studies highlighting the presence of similar 'prions' in the brains of affected people at post-mortem, a conclusive link between human consumption of contaminated bovine specified offal continues to be debated.

The only conclusive evidence for transmission to date has come from the field of surgical transmission, though this does not explain cases among people who have not undergone surgery. Duffy et al. (1974) reported transmission in one case by corneal transplantation, and Bernoulli et al. (1977) reported two further examples in young epileptic patients after using contaminated depth electrodes. Retrospective evidence now strongly incriminates neurological transmission in 3 of 8 patients included in Nevin et al.'s (1960) report (Will & Matthews, 1982).

Onset of CJD is usually between the ages of 40 and 60, but cases have been reported with onset at any adult age. The clinical features are very diverse from case to case, and were comprehensively reviewed by May (1968). A prodromal stage is usually described, lasting weeks or months and characterised by neurasthenic symptoms. The patient complains of fatigue, insomnia, anxiety and depression, and shows a gradual change towards mental slowness and unpredictability of behaviour. Intellectual deterioration or neurological defects become prominent. There may be ataxia of the cerebellar type, spasticity of limbs, with progressive paralysis, extrapyramidal rigidity, tremor or choreoathetoid movements, depending on the brain regions principally involved (Lishman, 1987). The course of CJD is more rapid than most other primary dementias, with over half of the patients dying within nine months and a great majority within two years. Death is usually preceded by a period of deepening coma, which lasts for several weeks.

Several sub-varieties of CJD have been described, depending upon the detailed neuropathological picture and partly upon the clinical features. Jones and Nevin (1954) and Nevin (1967) have labelled one such sub-variety 'subacute spongiform encephalopathy'. The age of onset is ten years later than that of the classical disease, and the beginning tends to be abrupt, without the usual prodromata. The course is extremely rapid, with a fatal ending after three to six months. Visual failure due to degeneration of the striate cortex has been a predominant feature in over a third of reported cases; irregular, shock-like jerks involving the entire body musculature also feature.

Another very rapid form has been named the 'ataxic form of subacute presenile polioencephalopathy' (Brownell & Oppenheimer, 1965). This is regarded as a nosological entity within the CJD group. It presents initially with rapidly progressive cerebellar ataxia, followed by dementia and abnormal motor movements in the form of rhythmic, myoclonic jerking, leading ultimately to generalised muscular rigidity. The principal findings at postmortem are selective degeneration of cells in the granular layer of the cerebellum, variable-status spongiosus, and cell loss and astrocytosis in the cortex, thalamus and striatum (Lishman, 1987). The amyotrophic form, which presents with muscle wasting, can sometimes run a relatively chronic course. This variety is unusual, in that it has not yet been proven to be transmissible to animals (Masters et al., 1970).

Multiple Sclerosis

Multiple sclerosis (MS) is a chronic, progressive disease, with symptoms that are often difficult to interpret and distinguish from other neurological disorders (Thompson, 1996a). The pathology of MS was first described over a hundred years ago (Miller & Hens, 1993), following its identification by the French neurologist Charcot in 1877. It has been described since as a chronic, degenerative disease, characterised by progressive demyelination of the central nervous system (Acorn & Andersen, 1990; McDonald, 1992). MS appears to have a higher incidence in the United States and Canada than in most countries (Acorn & Andersen, 1990); the onset being usually between the ages of 20 and 50 years (McDonald, 1992).

The common clinical features of MS include optic neuritis, sensory disturbances, spastic limb paresis, vertigo and balance problems, bowel disturbance, cerebellar symptoms and cognitive changes (Bennett, Dittmar & Raubach, 1991), such as memory disturbance (Peyser et al., 1980; Rao et al., 1984). Clinical research data for the diagnosis of MS have been established only since the 1960s (Poser, 1983; Schumacher, 1965), but with the advent of MRI of the central nervous system, characteristic lesions have become the main diagnostic investigation, with 95 per cent of clinically definite cases having characteristic MRI findings (Lee et al., 1991).

The combination of physical disability and psychological impairment (for example, dementia later on in the course of the disease) makes MS a difficult disease to treat, as well as to live with. Psychological adjustment (Lassen, 1990; Vanderplate, 1984) depends on a number of factors, including the number and type of support mechanisms in place (Gulick, 1994; Wineman et al., 1993), and the feeling of control (Wassem, 1991) as compared with empowerment (Miller, 1993) an individual with MS is experiencing. Various measures have been used to assess stressors and coping methods in people with MS; for example, the Barthel Index (Granger & Greer, 1976; Mahoney & Barthel, 1965) measures ability of patients with a neuromuscular disorder to care for themselves; the Jalowiec Coping Scale (Jalowiec & Powers, 1981) assesses coping styles, and the Multiple Sclerosis Stressor Scale (Buelow, 1991) evaluates stressors associated with MS. A combination of measures is often preferred, since the clinician or therapist needs to assess both cognitive and behavioural manifestations of MS (Mahler, 1992). Neuropsychological test batteries (Thompson, 1994a) are often used to establish the extent of presenting deficits, especially those that assess symptoms usually associated with dementia which are also typical of MS patients (Huber, Paulson & Shuttleworth, 1987).

The untreated course of MS is very variable, and up to a third of patients remain free of disability even after many years of relapsing disease activity (Thompson, 1996a). However, permanent disease occurs after MS enters a progressive phase (Heard, 1993). Encouraging results from clinical trials have shown that the drug Copolymer 1 seems to reduce flare-ups in MS by nearly 33 per cent (Maugh, 1995), but so far there is still no cure for this debilitating neurological disease.

Motor Neurone Disease

Motor neurone disease (MND), also known as 'amyotrophic lateral sclerosis' (ALS), is a progressive, non-inflammatory, degenerative and fatal disease of the nervous system. The disease affects the motor neurones in the brain and spinal cord. Degeneration causes weakness and wasting in the muscles supplying the limbs, face and throat, with consequent problems of thick speech and difficulty with chewing and swallowing (Beresford, 1995; Earll, Johnston & Mitchell, 1993).

Patients with MND progressively deteriorate over time; both the severity and speed are variable between patients. Death usually results from respiratory failure, with a mean survival time from diagnosis of four years: 20 per cent surviving over five years (Mulder & Howard, 1976), and 10 per cent surviving more than ten years. Onset can be at any age in adulthood, but peaks at 55–60 years (Harrison, 1983).

Researchers have reported varying degrees of psychological disturbance in MND patients, including dementia: for example, Peters, Wendell and Mulder (1978) found high scores on four scales of hypochondriasis, depression, hysteria and schizophrenia; Montgomery and Erickson (1987) found that 46 per cent of people with the condition had increased anxiety and depression, but that extreme depression was unrelated to severity of the disease. While various coping models for neurological conditions have been proposed (Leventhal, Nerenz & Steele, 1984; Nerenz & Leventhal, 1983), there is as yet neither a cure nor even significant, active, palliative treatment for MND.

Dementia Pugilistica

Dementia pugilistica (or 'punch drunk syndrome') is a clinical entity associated with the repeated head trauma sustained during boxing (Martland, 1928). In an extensive neuropathological study of 15 retired boxers, a characteristic pattern of brain damage was described (Corsellis, Bruton & Freeman-Brown, 1973). Dale et al. (1991) describe this pattern as damage to the septum pellucidum, scarring of the cerebellar and cerebral cortex, and loss of pigmented neurones in the substantia nigra regions of the brain. Neurofibrillary tangles, morphologically identical to those seen in Alzheimer's disease, were also seen in large numbers in cases of dementia pugilistica, particularly in the temporal lobe. However, another feature of Alzheimer's disease, neuritic senile plaques, were typically few or absent in cases of dementia pugilistica reviewed by Dale et al. (1991).

Alzheimer neurofibrillary tangles have been shown to contain epitopes of ubiquitin (a protein believed to play a role in the removal of abnormal and short-lived proteins from the cell) (Cole & Timiras, 1987; Mori, Kondo & Ihara, 1987; Perry et al., 1987). Dale et al. (1991) showed that ubiquitin is present in the neurofibrillary tangles of dementia pugilistica, as did Lennox et al. (1988). The significance of these findings is that ubiquitin has so far been the only protein consistently detected in inclusions associated with several neurodegenerative disorders, such as Lewy bodies in Parkinson's disease (Kuzuhara et al., 1988); anterior horn cell inclusions in motor neurone disease (Leigh et al., 1988; Lowe, Lennox & Jefferson, 1988; Kato et al., 1989); Pick bodies of Pick's disease (Leigh et al., 1989; Lowe, Blanchard & Morrell, 1988), in addition to the tangles of Alzheimer's disease and dementia pugilistica (Dale et al., 1991).

Brain damage to boxers often results from acceleration and deceleration of the brain within the skull, particularly rotational acceleration, resulting in the stretching of neurones and blood vessels by shearing forces, as well as linear acceleration, which produces focal lesions (Guterman & Smith, 1987). It is likely that neurofibrillary tangle formation occurs as a direct result of these damaging forces on neuronal processes (Dale et al., 1991). Head trauma may well be a factor in the development of Alzheimer's disease (Heyman et al., 1984), althoughgenetic susceptibility and environmental toxins currently appear to be favoured as putative causes (Dale et al., 1991).

Pseudodementia

Sometimes the clinical picture resembles organic dementia, yet there may be little or no indication of an organic cause. These types of disorders are termed 'pseudodementia', and include Ganser syndrome, hysterical pseudo-dementia, simulated dementia, depressive pseudodementia, and other rarer forms (Lishman, 1987). Often the distinction between organic dementia and pseudodementia is difficult to determine; as Lishman (1987) warns

> in the early stages of organic brain disease a patient may occasionally react in such a way that his dementia is suspected of being more apparent than real – in other words a pseudodementia may turn out in fact to be a 'pseudo-pseudodementia' (p. 404).

Ganser Syndrome

In 1898, Ganser described three prisoners who showed an unusual clinical picture which has been the focus of interest and controversy ever since (see Enoch, Trethowan & Barker, 1967; Whitlock, 1967). Typically, the patient's responses to questions are markedly inaccurate, and often absurdly so. However, they seem to betray a knowledge of the purpose of the question, and their close approximation to the correct answer implies that this knowledge is, at some level, available to the patient.

Lishman (1987) explains that approximate answers may be elicited in response to simple addition, counting, the naming of colours, or simple questions about everyday matters. Sometimes the patient may answer in a way quite contrary to the evidence before him/her: for example, stating that it is midnight when the sun is shining clearly through the window. The absurd responses are usually given with full deliberation and apparently serious intent, and false responses may be quite inconsistently interspersed with accurate answers.

All of Ganser's original patients also had prominent hallucinatory experiences, hysterical stigmata of various types, and showed evidence of fluctuating disturbance of consciousness. The abnormal mental state cleared suddenly, together with the hysterical conversion symptoms, and all of the patients were left with complete amnesia for the period of the illness.

Some researchers have debated the incidence of this syndrome, and this has led to the distinction between Ganser symptom and Ganser syndrome (Scott, 1965): the former is thought to be the most common, the latter extremely rare. Whitlock (1967) has suggested that for a diagnosis of the syndrome, in addition to 'approximate answers', there should be at least some evidence of impairment of consciousness, a sudden termination of the syndrome, and subsequent amnesia for the episode. McGrath and McKenna (1961) conclude that:

> The typical (approximate) answer is a compromise, simultaneously carrying on the original attempt to simulate and attempting to regain the lost reality by convincing both the patient himself and others that apprehension of the environment is still operating. The result of the message is a contradictory one, conveying 'I am insane, yet sane.' Hence the confusion in the diagnostic constructions put upon this relatively rare state. (p. 156).

The disorder would appear to rest principally on a complex psychogenic basis, in which hysterical mechanisms, or mechanisms closely allied to them, are largely responsible (Lishman, 1987). When organic or functional psychoses are seen in association with the Ganser manifestations, Lishman (1987) suggests that they have served principally as 'releasers', rather than as prime determinants of the condition.

Hysterical Pseudodementia

This is a type of pseudodementia mostly seen in people of low intellectual ability. The patient may be mute or monosyllabic in replies, or may be grossly incoherent and disorientated, failing on simple tests of cognitive function. The symptom of 'approximate answers' may be seen, but perseveration does not occur, and clear examples of concrete thinking will rarely be detected (Lishman, 1987).

Careful observation of the patient usually reveals that responses to commands are grossly inaccurate, with the patient producing an unconvincing and theatrical display of non-comprehension and inability to perform. According to Lishman (1987), the wrong reply or action may be followed later by the correct one, or patchy performance may fail to correspond to a hierarchy of increasing difficulty; also, the patient may be highly suggestible.

A comprehensive survey by Kennedy and Neville (1957) examined 74 patients with abrupt memory failure. They suggested that brain damage appeared to predispose to the development of primitive mental mechanisms of escape, or lower the threshold at which stress would bring them out:

> The flight was typically from simple situations to do with difficulties in marriage, bigamy or debt, but could also be from mental pain as in examples suffering from endogenous depression. (p. 428).

The great majority of their cases of psychogenic amnesia recovered within a few hours or several days when managed in the acute stage. In hysterical pseudodementia, there is often an antecedent history of severe personality instability, if not of previous hysterical conversion reactions. It is generally agreed that the whole reaction appears more superficial than in the Ganser syndrome, and that some elements of conscious malingering are more often detected. In addition, hysterical pseudodementia frequently runs a prolonged and relapsing course (unlike the typical, brief and sudden, spontaneous termination of Ganser episodes), particularly when the underlying conflicts are not treated or resolved.

Simulated Dementia

This is not commonly found, although in those rare instances when it is, motivation is usually gross (though sometimes not obvious to the examiner, or concealed), and close examination will often reveal signs inconsistent with a true diagnosis of dementia. Bluglass (1976) comments that such simulants usually fail to show the complete picture through ignorance, because they portray their own notion of dementia.

Benton and Spreen (1961) have found significant differences between groups of subjects simulating brain damage and patients with true brain damage. The researchers observed certain qualitative differences between their performances: the simulators made more errors of distortion than the patients in reproducing visual designs, and fewer errors of omission, perseveration and size. The malingerer, according to Kräupl-Taylor (1966), is likely to be anxiously on guard to avoid inconsistencies in his/her behaviour, and will become angry or upset and attempt to explain his/her errors when confronted with them. The self-deception of the person with pseudodementia often comprises a carelessness about the inconsistencies which he/she shows, and reactions may be bland, uncaring or even puzzled when brought to their attention.

Kennedy and Neville (1957) also felt that suggestibility may be another feature of difference between patients with psychogenic amnesia and true dementia. The former patients were found to be markedly suggestible during interview, though a small group who later confessed to malingering had hardly been suggestible at all. However, Lishman (1987) suggests that the simulator is much more likely than the hysterical patient to use his/her resources to defeat full inquiry, and to fail to co-operate in any close investigation. The final decision over diagnosis may rest on opinion about the patient's insight. For example, Farrell and Kaufman (1943) suggest that the clinician should be convinced that the individual is consciously aware of actions and requests and the motives for doing these. They should also be aware of the end result intended.

Depressive Pseudodementia

In this condition, the patient most commonly becomes slow to grasp essential aspects of the environment or about daily routines. Thinking is laboured, and behaviour becomes inefficient because of difficulty in concentrating or because of inner preoccupations. The impression of dementia is sometimes strengthened by the patient's decrepit appearance due to self-neglect and weight loss (Kiloh, 1961). Bourgeois, Hébert and Maisondieu (1970) presented several cases of apparent dementia in a setting of severe depression, all responding to electroconvulsive therapy (ECT) when antidepressant medication had failed.

The onset of endogenous depression is typically acute and recent, whereas that of dementia is insidious (Lishman, 1987). A careful history in depressive pseudodementia is therefore indicated, and may well reveal that such capacities as memory have not been affected up to the time of presentation of 'dementia'. Patients with depression will often complain of their cognitive abilities in a way that is quite different to those with dementia. Usually, these complaints are stated categorically, and sometimes forcefully so. Lishman (1987) comments that there is often a tendency for depressed patients to counter questions by 'don't know' responses, rather than the attempts to confabulate or make facile excuses for failure which are frequently observed in patients who are organically confused.

Other types of pseudodementia

Kiloh (1961) reports a rare case of hypomania which was initially mistaken for dementia. Distractibility in these patients is usually so severe that they cannot follow a coherent train of thought, and answers have an apparent randomness to them that initially deceives the observer into believing the patient to be grossly disorientated, with a very poor and failing memory.

Carney (1983) comments that episodes of mania in older people are particularly liable to produce a picture which at first sight suggests dementia. For instance, the overactivity is mistaken for agitation, and coherence and physical deterioration can combine to suggest an organic cerebral process. For these reasons, schizophrenia can also be mistaken for dementia. The poverty of ideas, blunting of emotion and unkempt appearance may strongly suggest dementia, and years of self-induced isolation and paranoid ideas might have led to a situation of chaos and disorganisation in their home (Roth, 1981).

However, the clinical distinction between schizophrenia and dementia usually rests on identifying first-rank symptoms of schizophrenic illness, or cardinal aspects of thought disorder. Similarly, identifying root causes or other traits, such as obsessive behaviour, may reveal obsessional, ruminative states or reactive depression instead of symptoms underlying dementia. In severe anxiety neurosis, the patient may come to focus on minor defects of memory, but may also be fearful of particular situations. Further investigation of the patient's background and history can usually help to tease out those symptoms that do not comfortably sit within the diagnosis of dementia.

Korsakoff's Psychosis

Albert (1978) has classified Korsakoff's psychosis among the subcortical dementias. Korsakoff's psychosis represents an end stage in a continuum of alcoholic deterioration. A number of different kinds of brain damage have been associated with the alcohol-related behavioural disturbances (Bolter & Hannon, 1980; Lishman, 1981). Alcohol (ethanol) acts as a central nervous system depressant, and has effects like those of some tranquillising and hypnotic drugs. Some of the data on brain atrophy suggest a selective shrinking of frontal and perhaps parietal lobe structures (Berglund & Risberg, 1980). Atrophy appears to be associated with the duration of problem drinking and the extent of cognitive deficit (Kroll et al., 1980; Lusins et al.,

1980). This atrophy appears to increase with age (Carlen, Wilkinson & Wortzman, 1981), and is thought to be due to the effects of alcohol itself (Walton, 1977).

Alcohol dementia may represent the end stage of the dementing process associated with alcohol-induced cerebral atrophy (Lezak, 1983). Chronic Korsakoff patients exhibit profound changes in affect and executive or control functions that may be more disabling and more representative of the psychological devastations of this disease than the memory impairments. Patients with this condition tend to be emotionally flat, lack the impulse to initiate activity, and if given a goal requiring more than an immediate, one-or two-step response, cannot organise, set into motion and carry through a plan of action to reach it (Biber, Butters & Rosen, 1981). For these reasons, it is sometimes difficult to assess such patients, especially since they often cannot give a social history or tell much about their current living conditions. However, information can sometimes be gained from informants, friends or relatives, or from past records, if kept.

Delirium Tremens

Delirium tremens is an acute disorder in which the most prominent symptoms are tremulousness, visual and other sensory hallucinations, and profound confusion and agitation that can lead to death from exhaustion. It is often associated with abrupt cessation of long-term drinking, but its exact aetiology remains unknown (Lishman, 1987).

Seizures and transient amnesic episodes (or 'blackouts') also occur in chronic alcoholics of long standing, usually during a heavy bout of drinking or soon after (Walton, 1977). Certain distinctive features, such as the tendency to confabulate (Howieson, 1980), gross memory defects (Butters & Cermak, 1974) and the usual state of affective blandness and passivity, clearly differentiate Korsakoff patients from other alcohol abusers. Intellectual deficits consistently appear on tasks involving functions associated with frontal lobe activity (Parsons, 1977; Talland, 1965; Tarter & Jones, 1971).

Difficulties in maintaining a cognitive set, impersistence, decreased flexibility in thinking, defective visual searching behaviour, deficient motor inhibition, perseveration, loss of spatial and temporal orientation, and impaired ability to organise perceptuomotor responses and synthesise spatial elements characterise the behaviour of chronic alcoholics (Lezak, 1983). Performance by Korsakoff patients on well-structured, untimed tests of familiar, usually overlearned material (such as the vocabulary and arithmetic sub-tests of the Wechsler Adult Intelligence Scale) hold up, unlike scores on tests that require speed, visuoperceptual, spatial organisation, or short-term memory, which are very poor.

Patients with Korsakoff's psychosis usually demonstrate new learning, but may exhibit difficulty with retrieval; this is due to thalamic and mammillary body lesions. Korsakoff's psychosis has been shown to be due to a nutritional deficiency of vitamin B$_1$ (thiamine) (Lishman, 1981; Walton, 1977). The diet of chronic alcoholics, particularly during periods of binge drinking, often fails to meet the body's thiamine needs.

Habit-forming Drugs and Toxins

A number of studies point to personality changes in heavy users of marijuana or hashish. The most commonly described characteristics are affective blunting, mental and physical sluggishness, apathy, restlessness, some mental confusion, and defective recent memory (Lezak, 1983). Evans (1975) reported enlarged ventricles in the brains of youthful marijuana smokers, but these findings have been debated by others (Lishman, 1987). Long-term brain damage or dementia is still supposition in long-standing users of marijuana.

Particular industrial toxins, such as organic solvents used in house paint, may also cause neuropsychological effects, especially in people whose occupations necessitate regular exposure to these components. It is also known that farm-workers exposed to sheep dip containing organophosphates have presented with dementia-like symptoms, though some researchers have found little change in brain atrophy over time – for example, inhouse-painters after a two-year follow-up study (Bruhn et al., 1981).

Mikkelsohn (1980) and others (Gregersen, Middelsen & Klausen, 1978) found that painters and other industrial workers exposed to organic solvents suffer conditions of debilitating dementia at a higher than normal rate in their middle years. They raise the question of whether such exposure may be a possible consequence of presenile dementia (Gregersen, Middelsen & Klausen, 1978). More long-term studies need to be evaluated for these suggestions to be confirmed, but perhaps more caution should be exercised when working in these possibly hazardous occupational areas.

Differential Diagnosis

Several studies have warned of the difficulties of diagnosis, especially in the early stages of dementia, as subtle personality changes are easily overlooked (Mohanaruban, Sastry & Finucane, 1989). However, some distinctions can be made between the presenting clinical features of common conditions; for example, the onset of 'acute confusion' is usually sudden and of short duration; 'dementia' (chronic confusion) has a slow and steadily progressive onset, while 'depression' (pseudodementia) may take place over a number of discrete episodes. Sufferers of depression seem generally to have insight into their condition, often complaining of an impaired memory; on the other hand, sufferers of dementia and acute confusion seem not to have any insight into the problem (Mohanaruban, Sastry & Finucane, 1989). Other forms of pseudodementia include hypomania, which can occasionally produce a picture which is mistaken for dementia. Pseudodementias are basically conditions in which a clinical picture resembles organic dementia, yet physical disease proves to be little (if at all) responsible for the presenting symptoms (see Katzman & Karasu, 1975).

Testimony regarding the difficulties encountered in the differential diagnosis of dementia and depression is abundant in the literature (Benedict & Nacoste, 1990). Reviews of follow-up diagnostic studies cite evidence of dementia being misdiagnosed as depression (for example, Feinberg & Goodman, 1984; Fisman, 1985; Reding, Haycox & Blass, 1985); they also contain examples of the more commonly occurring phenomenon where depression is initially misdiagnosed as dementia (for example, Garcia, Reding & Blass, 1981; Kaszniak, 1986). There is also another possibility: the coexistence of depression and dementia. The diagnostic confusion and uncertainty that surround these two disorders is also reflected by neuropsychological studies which have found overlapping performance of demented and depressed patients (La Rue, 1982), and by papers demonstrating the potential for age-related biases when making diagnostic and treatment decisions concerning dementia and depression (for example, Perlick & Atkins, 1984; Gatz & Pearson, 1988).

Different opinions have been expressed concerning the nature of the depression observed in cases of Alzheimer-type dementia. Clinicians have conventionally viewed depression as a reactive phenomenon, more likely to occur during the early stages of the dementia when a modicum of insight remains (Zarit, 1980; MacInnes, 1983; Mahendra, 1985). A similar explanation has been offered for the depression that accompanies multi-infarct dementia (Hachinski, 1983), which is characterised by the occurrence of many small infarcts, primarily caused by blockage or rupture to the numerous small vessels that serve the brain tissue. The decreasing level of depression over the course of these two types of dementia has been contrasted to the rising level of depression sometimes observed over the course of 'subcortical' dementias (see Lishman, 1987) stemming from disorders such as Parkinson's disease and Huntington's disease (Shuttleworth, Huber & Paulson, 1987). Although the DSM-III-R (APA, 1987) does not directly address this topic, it seems to imply a similar interpretation by stating that marked anxiety and depressive reactions may occur when Alzheimer-type dementia is mild. However, DSM-IV (APA, 1994) recognises the frequent coexistence of depression in the diagnostic criteria presented.

Further Reading

Burish, T. & Bradley L.A. (1983), Coping with Chronic Disease: Research and Applications, London: Academic Press.

Jorm, A.F. (1987), Understanding Senile Dementia, London: Chapman & Hall.

McGowin, D.F. (1993), Living in the Labyrinth: A Personal Journey Through the Maze of Alzheimer's, San Francisco: Elder Books.

Miller, E. & Morris, R. (1993), The Psychology of Dementia, Chichester: John Wiley.

Rao, S.M., Hammeke, T.A., McQuillen, M.P., Khatri, O.O., et al. (1984), 'Memory disturbance in chronic progressive multiple sclerosis', Archives of Neurology, 41: 625–31.

Rao, S.M., Huber, S.J. & Bornstein, R.A. (1992), 'Emotional changes with multiple sclerosis and Parkinson's disease', Journal of Consulting & Clinical Psychology, 60, 3: 369–78.

Wattis, J. & Martin, C. (1993), Practical Psychiatry of Old Age, London: Chapman & Hall.

Chapter 3

Memory Disorders

Probably one of the most well known reports of a head injury is that of Phineas Gage, the foreman of a road construction gang in the USA in 1848, when a tamping iron was driven through his skull following an explosion. He survived, but the damage to his frontal lobes led to a considerable change in personality, from being a considerate, efficient and well-balanced man to being obstinate, profane and showing little consideration for others (Haste & Gregory,1993).

Very often, the effects of a head injury are more subtle; forgetfulness is common and can cause distress as well as inconvenience not only to the patient but also to the patient's family and friends. Post-traumatic amnesia (PTA) is the time from impact until recovery of continuous memory (Giles & Clark-Wilson, 1993). Psychosocial recovery (McKinlay & Brooks, 1984) following severe head injury can often take much longer. For example, many patient with head injuries become depressed, making it difficult to assess the extent of their remaining abilities. Anxiety too may follow and is often the result of confusion following unconsciousness or frequently, a fear of not being able to perform the tasks (for example, activities of daily living) that they were able to perform competently prior to the accident.

Intact Memory

A distinction is commonly drawn between a short-term memory system of limited capacity, a few items at most and a storage of seconds, and a long-term system of perhaps limitless capacity, and indefinite storage time (Atkinson & Shiffrin, 1968). Short-term memory, now elaborated to the concept of working memory, (Baddeley, Wilson & Watts, 1995), is the system that enables a new telephone number to be remembered while dialling it - so long as there is no distraction. Long-term memory allows one to remember a familiar telephone number from day to day and year to year (Collerton, 1993). This terminology differs from commonplace use where short-term memory is taken to be the memory for the preceding hours, days or months, and long-term memory to be memory for many years in the past.

It is now believed that there are four processing stages involved in memory: registration, encoding, storage and retrieval. For information to be stored in memory, it must first be attended to or registered. Encoding is the process whereby this information may be semantically encoded or phonologically encoded (Baddeley, 1978), that is, encoded in terms of meaning or sound respectively. Storage is the process by which information is maintained in memory. It is widely accepted that different types of knowledge appear to be stored differently, so that, for example, knowing what a person ate for lunch (episodic memory) would be stored differently from knowing that the word 'lunch' means a mid-day meal (semantic memory). Cohen and Squire (1981) have subsumed these terms under 'declarative memory' and reserve a further definition, termed 'procedural memory', for skills and routines including some types of sensory memory (for example, knowing how to ride a motorbike is a procedural memory while knowing how the engine works is declarative). These functional definitions of memory have practical applications for therapists and are also more simplistic than earlier definitions.

Retrieval is the process by which information is made available from memory and is thought to be dependent upon a number of factors, such as the closeness in which conditions are matched at encoding and retrieval (Tulving, 1979) and the strategy used for retrieving memorised information (Roediger III & Blaxton, 1987).

Types of Memory Disorders

A look at the case histories of patients examined for memory impairments has shown that people's memory for events is very selective (Thompson, 1995). Selective memory is difficult to explain but, generally, people remember only certain details of an event (Eich, 1984) and this is often not under conscious control as in the case of the brain-injured person. People experiencing traumatic events sometimes repress distressing memories. The process used here is blocking the retrieval of information rather than preventing information from being memorised in the first place (Terr, 1994). Boring or over-complicated information is also selectively ignored and not retained, but this may also be carried out at a conscious level by intact individuals (without brain injury). It is a constant battle, therefore, for therapists and clinicians to seek out stimulating information while still achieving an objective assessment of patient's memory functioning.

A number of different amnesiac conditions following head injury have been reported, for example, transient epileptic amnesia (Kapur,

1993) and fugue states (Kapur, 1991). A distinction has also been made between lost memories for childhood events and occurrences prior to the accident, that is, retrograde amnesia, and those events and memories lost following the accident, that is, anterograde amnesia (O'Connor *et al.,* 1992; Kapur *et al.,* 1996a). However, PTA, as described by Russell (1971), is sometimes difficult to determine. For example, in severe global anterograde amnesia, day-to-day memories may never return; therefore, PTA effectively becomes indefinite. Other causes for 'not remembering' include perceptual and attention deficits. Focused attention, rigidity of thinking or inadequate organisation or prioritisation of material can lead to inappropriate selection of material to retain. Information-processing deficits are also common among brain-injured patients.

Another problem that therapists face with headinjured patients is the classification of the severity of amnesia. Currently, there is no generally accepted classification except for a division in terms of performance on standardised tests of memory (Mayes, 1986). But this has limited value for real life situations. Gordon (1987) has emphasised the importance of knowledge learnt in one setting and the patient's ability to generalise this knowledge to other settings. This seems to be a more useful measure of amnesiac severity as well as the uncontested usefulness in terms of therapeutic rehabilitation.

Three levels of generalisation have been distinguished as follows:

1. The results of training on a task should generalise from one session to the next, as well as to alternative forms of the training material.
2. Improvement should generalise to memory tests both similar to and different from the task that was trained.
3. Improvement should generalise from the particular task to everyday living.

Glisky, Schacter and Tulving (1986) have warned that some patients with amnesia have great difficulty in level 3 generalisation. This can lead to 'hyperspecific learning' where recall can only take place if the conditions of learning are exactly recreated.

Memory Problems Associated with Dementia

Memory disorders as a result of Alzheimer's disease or vascular dementia may have very different presentations. The reader is referred to Thompson (1997) for a critical discussion and review of the literature.

In recent years, people with Alzheimer's disease have been helped by the advances of so-called 'antidementia' medication (eg *Reminyl, Aricept,* and *Exelon)* which has shown promising results for people who have been diagnosed early on (NCCHTA, 2001; Thompson, MacDonald & Coates, 2001).

Further Reading

Kapur N (1994) *Memory Disorders in Clinical Practice.* Hove, Lawrence Erlbaum.

Miller E (1992) Psychological approaches to the management of memory impairments. *British Journal of Psychiatry, 160, 1-6.*

NCCHTA - National Coordinating Centre for Health Technology Assessment (2001) *Clinical and CostEffectiveness of Donepezil, Rivastigmine and Galantamine for Alzheimer's Disease: A Rapid and Systematic Review.* Southampton: National Coordinating Centre for Health Technology Assessment.

Thompson SBN (2002) Memory decline, Alzheimer's disease and vascular dementia: The clinical picture. *Journal of Cognitive Rehabilitation,* 20; 2: 12-18.

Thompson SBN, MacDonald J & Coates TD (2001) Improving visual memory with Aricept (Donepezil Hydrochloride, E2020) in mild-to-moderate Alzheimer's disease. *Clinical Gerontologist,* 24; 12, 55-73.

Thompson SBN & Watson F (2001) `Hollywood Wives': Education and support for spouses of inpatients with dementia. *Journal of Dementia Care,* 9; 2: 38.

Chapter 4

Learning Disability and Dementia

Definition of 'Learning Disability'

Two per cent of the UK population (over 1 million people) have learning disabilities, the majority of them mild. In 1991, 4,500 babies were born with severe learning disabilities (6 in 1,000 live births); more people with learning disabilities are male (54 per cent) than female (46 per cent) (Mental Health Foundation, 1993).

'Learning disability' (formerly known as 'mental handicap') is a very broad term and has been used to describe people with an intelligence quotient (IQ) below 70. Both terms commonly describe people who, in fact, may have a range of difficulties, including approaches to problem-solving, co-ordination difficulties, problems with speech or comprehension, cognitive delay, or slowness or inability to perform daily routines, such as hygiene or feeding (Thompson, 1993a). The range or number of difficulties an individual may have can be very large, or equally, very small. Increasingly, therefore, it has been useful to state a person's abilities rather than emphasising their negative disabilities. With the promotion of community living, definitions of learning disability have come to include the extent of a person's ability to live alone, or his or her 'independence'. A useful working definition, taken from Thompson (1993b), has been adopted for several studies:

> A person with a learning disability is someone who is, to a varying degree, dependent on others for their living needs because of a cognitive impairment resulting from hereditary abnormalities or directly following (or during) birth. They may (or may not) also have associated physical/sensory/behavioural/medical disabilities' (p. 195).

Definition of Down's Syndrome

Down's syndrome (previously termed 'mongolism') is one of the most frequently observed forms of learning disability (for example, Moody & Moody, 1992). The term 'Down's syndrome' is used more often clinically, and was first described by Langdon Down as a separate entity in 1866 (Down, 1866) and independently in the same year by Seguin (1866). Seguin referred to the disorder as 'furfuraceous cretinism', emphasising an assumed relationship to cretinism, while Down, struck by some aspects of the physiognomy of the patients which were superficially similar to those of people in outer Mongolia, called it 'Mongolian idiocy'. Thankfully, today people with such disorders are more commonly referred to by their first names, thus recognising the fact that there is a person behind such stigmatising labels!

A characteristic of Down's syndrome is the presence of an extra gene on chromosome 21 (trisomy 21) (Shermann et al., 1991). Often the person has developmental delays (Maclean et al., 1991), sometimes a slightly larger head circumference (Palmer et al., 1992), and language difficulties, especially with ageing (Young & Kramer, 1991). Down's syndrome has been the focus of much research and controversy (Barr, 1990). Because of increased longevity (Day, 1985; Eyman et al., 1987; Eyman, Call & White, 1991), individuals with Down's syndrome are living long enough to be at risk of a host of age-related diseases (Young & Kramer, 1991), for example, pre-senile dementia (Wisniewski et al., 1983).

Link between Down's Syndrome and Alzheimer's Disease

An association between Down's syndrome and dementia was first noted by Fraser and Mitchell in 1876, but it was not until 1929 that Struwe described the characteristic senile plaques of Alzheimer's disease in the brains of individuals with Down's syndrome. Jervis (1948) and Verhaart and Jelgersma (1952) described clinical deterioration associated with Alzheimer-like changes at post-mortem in a number of people with Down's syndrome; subsequent research focused on establishing similarities between the neuropathological changes in the brains of elderly Down's syndrome individuals and the senile plaques, neurofibrillary tangles and granulovascular degeneration characteristic of Alzheimer's disease. By the 1960s, the link between the two disorders was clearly established, and it was agreed that all people with Down's syndrome over the age of 35 have the neuropathological features of Alzheimer's disease.

Learning Disability and Dementia

Alzheimer's disease (Heston, 1977). However, there is still debate over whether or not people with Down's syndrome also present with typical clinical features of Alzheimer's disease (Roper & Williams, 1980), since many such individuals maintain good physical and mental health into their forties and fifties (see Sylvester, 1984; St Clair & Blackwood, 1985).

Interest in the relationship between Alzheimer's disease and Down's syndrome has been stimulated by discoveries localising two distinct Alzheimer's disease markers to chromosome 21. First, the gene encoding the precursor protein which, in some processed form, gives rise to the amyloid deposits in Alzheimer's disease, is found on chromosome 21 (Kang et al., 1987). Second, a marker has been identified on chromosome 21 which is linked to within 15 centrimorgans (a distance spanning 300–600 genes or 15 million base pairs) of a site associated with an autosomal dominant form of Alzheimer's disease (St George-Hyslop et al., 1987).

Arguments in favour of some kind of connection have been advanced for some time (for example, Prosser, 1989), but evidence from some studies also calls into doubt such a definitive connection; for example, it is suggested that the amyloidogenic gene on chromosome 21 is not identical to the Alzheimer's gene, despite the widespread presence of amyloid material in the senile plaques and neurofibrillary tangles (Curran & Wattis, 1989). This might imply that the picture reflected in Down's syndrome may be of a different brain process to that evidenced in people who have Alzheimer's disease.

Difficulties in Identifying Dementia

It should be noted that, like the general population, people with learning disabilities can develop any of the different types of dementia – multi-infarct, arteriosclerotic or parenchymatous (such as Alzheimer's disease). As with the general population, these different diseases have different courses: for example, step-wise versus insidious decline when comparing multi-infarct dementia with Alzheimer's disease. Currently, more is known about the link between Down's syndrome and Alzheimer's disease.

Although there is little definitive evidence of a family history of Alzheimer's disease in sufferers, an assumed inheritance of Alzheimer's disease within families has been reported in a few studies (for example, Heston et al., 1981; Whalley et al., 1982; Breitner & Folstein, 1984). However, these studies are difficult to compare and have been criticised for having poor fol-low-up of subjects or using different criteria for the diagnosis of dementia (for example, Roth, 1955; Larsson, Sjögren & Jacobson, 1963; McKusick, 1983). Studies of twins have been used to try to disentangle the roles of environment and genetics. In one such study, the incidence of dementia for monozygotic twins was found to be less than for dizygotic twins (Deary & Whalley, 1988). Thus, although genetic factors are important, environmental factors seem to play an essential role.

A number of difficulties arise when attempting to assess people with a learning disability, whether or not they possess the signs associated with dementia. For example, many of these clients have limited or poorly-developed language, poor comprehension, apraxia or agnosia, or suffer from depressive illness (see Yapa & Roy, 1990; Cooper & Collacott, 1993), or other psychiatric disabilities (Moss, Goldberg & Patel, 1991). They may have specific physical disabilities, such as incontinence, abnormal reflexes, or behavioural problems (for example, inappropriate behaviour, stereotyped movements or pronounced anxiety) that make conventional psychological testing awkward or even impossible. These clients may simply manifest the processes of normal ageing (Thase et al., 1983; Hewitt, Carter & Jancar, 1985; Gath, 1986; Zigman et al., 1987; Hogg, Moss & Cooke, 1988a).

In some neuropathological studies of Down's syndrome, it has been suggested that the present diagnostic criteria and clinical signs of Alzheimer's disease are easily applicable (Reid & Aungle, 1974; Reid, Mahoney & Aungle, 1978), while others argue that the signs of deterioration associated with ageing in Down's syndrome need to be clarified before the diagnosis of Alzheimer's disease can be generally accepted (Burger & Vogel, 1973; Ellis, McCulloch & Corley, 1974; Sylvester, 1984). The major difficulty in applying criteria is the underlying learning disability. As Levinson, Friedman and Stamps (1955) have commented, there is great variation in the developmental theories and in the IQs of people with Down's syndrome (and other learning disabilities), 30 per cent scoring less than 20 points, 65 per cent between 20 and 50, and 5 per cent between 50 and 65 (Breg, 1977). These impose great restraints on the application and interpretation of conventional test procedures (for example, Moulin, 1980; Jones, 1987; Atkinson, 1991a): failure or poor performance might indicate dementia or an underlying disability. Clearly, these restrictions would not apply if the 'intelligence' of this client population was evenly distributed throughout age groups.

When considering these issues, other questions are raised. For instance, are the associated changes in behaviour present but undetected in people with Down's syndrome due to poor institutional environments? To complicate this further, it also seems likely that there is an increased prevalence of epilepsy with age in sufferers of Alzheimer's disease (for example, Sourander & Sjögren, 1970; Veall, 1974; Crapper et al., 1975; Tangye, 1979). Making the distinction between the effects of long-term epilepsy and types of brain damage on cerebral function can often be a difficult process (Thompson & Morgan, 1996; Thompson, North & Pentland, 1992).

Although a high proportion of individuals with Down's syndrome develop the neuropsychological changes of Alzheimer's disease, only a proportion develop the definite signs of deterioration and have the clinical features characteristic of the later stages of Alzheimer's disease. It is also often difficult to discriminate between pre- or perinatal brain damage (for example, meningitis, anoxia) in association with normal ageing (see Gath, 1986) and those considered to be the result of a dementing process, such as multi-infarcts or Alzheimer's disease (for example, Haxby, 1989). The situation is more complicated in people with a learning disability when there are other confounding variables, such as the long-term effects of institutional living, communication and comprehension difficulties, and the lack of a pre-morbid intelligence quotient, since intellectual deficits may have originated from birth.

The paradox between unequivocal neuropathological findings and limited clinical evidence of dementia, particularly in Down's syndrome, has been partly resolved by the use of specific neuropsychological assessments to detect age-related deficits (for example, Dalton, Crapper & Schlotterer, 1974; Wisniewski et al., 1978; Miniszek, 1983; Wisniewski et al., 1983; Dalton, 1992), but conclusive evidence to distinguish clinical features of dementia from normal ageing in people with Down's syndrome is still not available.

Combining cognitive tests with other measures of Alzheimer's pathology (for example, computerised axial tomography scans – see Schapiro et al., 1987) may reveal more distinctive early clinical indicators of deterioration. Indeed, St Clair and Blackwood's (1985) finding that evoked potential latency in those with Down's syndrome increased significantly earlier in life than normal controls may provide this early indication when correlated with cognitive test results. In the absence of such technology, conventional psychological techniques must be used, but careful selection and possible modification of test batteries becomes necessary when assessing people with learning disabilities.

Social and Cultural Differences

In 1994, the 25th anniversary of the first statement of the principle of normalisation in the human service literature was celebrated. Normalisation (also termed 'social role valorization') (Wolfensberger & Kugel, 1969) is a complex term covering a number of important different areas of living skills. Broadly, it can be defined in three ways.

Values

Normalisation is based on the belief that people with learning disabilities should be socially accepted and valued, with the same rights as other non-learning-disabled people who live in the mainstream of society as valued and respected citizens. Within different cultures, there are specific rights and societal positions. For example, the Chinese community is regarded as having a high respect for its elders, especially the grandparents, who have a key role in decisions and life in the family. Little is known about the integration of people with learning disabilities in specific cultures, but it is suspected that this varies greatly, with poorer care being associated with countries that have poor economies or poorly-run health services.

Health and Social Services

Normalisation also has implications for the design and delivery of services to people with learning disabilities. There have been several changes in attitude over the years about the delivery and type of services, and management implications. For example, Local Based Hospital Units (LBHUs) used to be the chosen housing for people with learning disabilities moving from large institutions into ward-type accommodation, often comprising 20- or 25-bed, dormitory-style rooms. A move away from LBHUs to smaller 'group homes' of four or five residents followed, with an increasing emphasis on 'normal' accommodation, such as houses or bungalows in ordinary housing areas. Older people, with or without learning disabilities, have often been rehoused according to financial constraints; some people moving from 'long-stay' institutions have been re-located to geographical areas previously unknown to themselves, but with such tentative links as being their original place of birth. Clearly, this is inhumane, and people with learning disabilities deserve the rights given to everyone in choosing where to live.

Relationships

Normalisation includes views and feelings about other people, and how people with learning disabilities interact at a personal level. It is also about the rights of older people with learning disabilities, and includes such rights as expressing their sexuality (see Thompson, 1990, 1994b).

In 1985, Somerset Social Services Department and the local health authority put together an ambitious strategy (Turnbull, 1993): first, to establish social services as the lead agency in this field, and second, to close three hospitals for people with learning disabilities. The benefits for former residents, whose lifestyles were now more ordinary, and who were rightly proud of their achievements, was highlighted in an evaluation conducted by the University of Kent (Somerset County Council, 1992) that showed these new arrangements to be superior.

Around the UK, other agencies have evaluated their services following earlier recommendations from the Jay Report (Jay, 1979) and Cullen Report (Cullen, 1991). Services for people with learning disabilities in Gwent were provided for ten years within the framework of the All Wales Strategy and All Wales Specialist Nurse Group (1992), and previously, the Welsh Office (1983). According to Kay (1993), the Briggs Committee (Briggs, 1972) took considerable discussion to suggest a new role for mental handicap nursing in 1972. It seems that any change to existing services takes time and entails convincing the relevant decision-makers. Certainly, before long we will be faced with the situation of caring for older people with learning disabilities and with providing them with equivalent care to our existing older population. However, rather than training people with specialist roles, for example, specialist nurses, Cox (1993) advocates that we should be focusing on meeting the various needs of people with learning disabilities; then, the role of the nurse will become evident. This seems to make sense so long as our specialism-trained staff are not lost or our special skills substituted by generic workers with rather diluted skills.

Social Rejection

Rejection comes in many forms. Sometimes it is overt, such as bullying in playgrounds by children; at other times it is more subtle, such as prejudice in job selection or favouritism during the delegation of duties. Older people with learning disabilities can face many forms of social rejection, not only because of the way they look (for example, if they have Down's syndrome) (Gath, 1986), but because of the way they talk (Bayles & Boone, 1982; Hartley, 1982; Young & Kramer, 1991) or act (Reid, 1982). The fact of increased survival of people with Down's syndrome has been well documented (Fryers, 1986), but less is known about, for example, how positive attitudes may allow children with learning disabilities to be given human value in the community. Hopefully, this would then continue through to adulthood and older age.

Older people without learning disabilities are often socially rejected
if they have socially undesirable ailments; having a learning disability
in addition may exaggerate this rejection. As Fryers (1986) suggests,
as treatments for serious causes of vulnerability are successful and
absorbed into common medical practices, difficult problems become
more visible and compelling. Hence, people with learning disabilities
and obvious (and perhaps antisocial) problems present many
difficulties for carers because of society's 'policy' of rejection, as well
as the medical conditions, which themselves present demands upon
carers.

Stereotyping is very much to blame for rejecting people with
certain conditions of all ages. Contrary to the stereotype of the silent
and withdrawn person with autism, for example, the person with
Asperger's syndrome may have fluent language. Described by the
Austrian psychiatrist, Hans Asperger (1944; 1968; 1979), confusion
followed his use of the term 'autistic psychopathy' to describe this
population. This led to misunderstanding because of the popular
tendency to equate psychopathy with sociopathic behaviour (Wing,
1981). Hydrocephalus, phenylketonuria (Medical Research Council,
1993; Pueschel, Yeatman & Hum, 1977; Thompson, 1995b) and
self-injurious behaviour (Repp, Felce & Barton, 1988) are additional
conditions associated with learning disabilities, and each places
increased demands upon carers and upon peers in terms of social
acceptance.

As longevity becomes more prevalent, these problems will also
appear more frequently in the emerging older age group of learning-
disabled people. It would seem that having fought the battle for
society's acceptance, at some level, of people with learning disabilities,
the battle for acceptance of people with a range of additional problems
at an older age has only just begun.

Further Reading

Cutler, N.R. (1985), 'Alzheimer's disease and Down's syndrome: New
    insights', *Annals of Internal Medicine*, 103: 556–78.
Fryers, T. (1986), 'Survival in Down's syndrome', *Journal of Mental
    Deficiency Research*, 30: 101–10.
Seltzer, M. & Krauss, M. (1987), *Aging and Mental Retardation:
    Extending the Continuum*, Washington, D.C.: American Association
    on Mental Deficiency.
Thase, M.E. (1982), 'Reversible dementia in Down's syndrome',
    Journal of Mental Deficiency Research, 26: 111–13.
Thompson, S.B.N. (1993b), *Eating Disorders: A Guide for Health*

Professionals, London: Chapman & Hall, 194–240.

Wisniewski, K.E., Howe, J., Williams, D.G. & Wisniewski, H.M. (1978), 'Precocious ageing and dementia in patients with Down's syndrome', *Biological Psychiatry*, 13: 619–27.

Wolfensberger, W. & Kugel, R. (1969), *Changing Patterns in Residential Services for the Mentally Retarded*, Washington, D.C.: President's Committee on Mental Retardation.

Zigman, W.B., Schupf, N., Lubin, R.A. & Silverman, W.P. (1987), 'Premature regression of adults with Down's syndrome', American *Journal of Mental Deficiency*, *92,* 2: 161-8.

PART II
Coping with Memory Problems

Chapter 5

How to Treat Memory Problems

Following assessment, various treatment strategies may be explored. Dementia *per se* cannot be corrected but some aspects of cognitive functioning can be maintained or improved with re-training. The majority of strategies tried and tested and reported in the clinical literature have been mainly for treating problems of *declarative memory*.

While repetitive practice seems to affect 'knowing' items, it has been shown to be ineffective for remembering items (Gardiner, Gawlik & Richardson-Klavehn, 1994). Elaborative rehearsal and specific mnemonic strategies (Richardson, 1992) have been used to help patients with impaired declarative memory function. Some approaches have aimed to capitalise on the commonly spared procedural memory in patients with amnesia; for example, Glisky and Schacter (1988) have used employable data-processing skills with people with dense amnesias, though learning was slower than normal. In contrast, external aids have been used in numerous settings in an attempt to reduce the handicapping effects of amnesia. Both approaches have their merits and their successes, and the patient's individual needs as well as the most comfortable working style for the therapist should dictate the memory strategy chosen. However, wherever possible, the therapist should seek others' expertise in order to match the approach to the individual patient's abilities and requirements.

It should be borne in mind that dementia may involve an insidious and progressive deterioration (for example, as in Alzheimer's disease), which will also lead to effects on memory functioning and capacity. A step-wise deterioration (such as that seen in multi-infarct dementia) may produce a different pattern of memory failure over time. Hence, 'compensatory' versus 'restorative' approaches to memory re-training will be more useful.

The majority of strategies have been carried out for problems of declarative memory. Whilst repetitive practice seems to affect *knowing* items, it has been shown to be ineffective for *remembering* items (Gardiner, Gawlik & Richardson-Klavehn, 1994). Elaborative rehearsal and also specific mnemonic strategies (Richardson, 1992) have been used to help patients with impaired declarative memory function. Some approaches have been aimed at capitalising on the commonly spared procedural memory in patients with amnesia; for example, Glisky & Schacter (1988) have used employable data-processing skills with people with dense amnesia, although learning was slower than normal. In contrast, external aids have been used in numerous settings in an attempt to reduce the handicapping effects of amnesia.

Both approaches have their merits. The patient's individual needs as well as the most comfortable working style of the therapist should dictate the memory strategy chosen although, whenever required and possible, the therapist should seek others' expertise in order to meet the individual abilities and requirements of the patient. Both interventions depend upon the timing of the rehabilitation; the types of strategy used prior to the injury and the effectiveness of the person's current strategies; the methods appropriate for the patient's recovery; and the other deficits the patient is left with following brain injury.

External Aids and Tips

The following have been found to be useful aids, mainly for prompting patients to remember items or appointments (Kurleycheck, 1983; Hanley & Lusty, 1984):

1. Keeping a calendar handy the can be changed for the day.
2. Keeping photographs of familiar people on view.
3. Labelling the doors of all rooms.
4. Using a notice board to display information to be remembered.
5. Keeping a clock with a large clear dial on view.
6. Leaving everyday possessions in handy places, always keeping them in the same location.
7. Keeping furniture in the same place.
8. Making a list of things to do so that they can be ticked off as they are done (by patient or helper).
9. Leaving out things that are needed.
10. When going out, leaving the address on a piece of paper to inform friends/ relatives.
11. Sticking to a routine as far as possible.
12. Setting out things to do in order of priority.

Other useful ways of prompting a poor memory include: using memo stickers; writing on the back of one's hand (!); using a wristwatch with an alarm; and electronic memory aids such as personal organisers. Various attempts have been made to evaluate memory in everyday life (Crook & Larrabee, 1992). Findings from studies have shown that a simple system of prompting that helps carers and relatives as well as patients is most useful, such as a booklet or list of memory tips, since many patients need prompting to use the memory prompts themselves (Collerton, 1993).

Internal Strategies

There are a number of strategies that may be learned and internalized. These are referred to as 'internal strategies' as compared with those that are 'external' such as using prompts or labels to help remember things that tend to be forgotten.

The following strategies have been shown by therapists and clinicians to be useful for some patients with a failing memory. The subheadings relate to items often forgotten by patients.

Problems Remembering

- **What you have read**

Sometimes you may forget a story that you have just read in a magazine or newspaper, or the gist of what has just been read in a book or in a magazine article. A useful strategy is the PQRST method (Robertson-Tchabo, Hausman & Arenberg, 1976; Glasgow, Zeiss & Barrera, 1977):

P is for Preview: Read the story quickly so you know roughly what it is about.
Q is for Question: Ask yourself something about the story
R is for Read: Read the story again, more slowly this time, and try to answer the questions as you do this.
S is for State: Say to yourself (or out loud) what the story is about.
T is for Test: Now, answer those questions again.

If the PQRST method is practised several times, it gets easier to use and memory often improves.

- **Words and sentences**

Some people have particular difficulty in remembering what words go together whether in speech or when writing them down.

Try to put the words you want to remember in an unusual sentence. Practise saying the sentence. If you want to remember pairs of words (for example, `up and down) then picture them in your mind: a person going up and down a staircase or on a see-saw, or any image that is clear for you to remember. When you want to remember the words, try to remember the picture (Crovitz, Harvey & Home, 1979).

- **Past memories**

Some things can trigger people's past memories. There may be certain strong associations or links that are made at the time of remembering or when the information is stored, such as tastes, smells, colours or textures felt. Presenting yourself with such items can sometimes bring back memories and sensation are often re-experienced. Listening to a record or reading out a poem or story remembered from childhood may bring back childhood memories (Burnside, 1990; Kovach, 1990).

- **People's names**

Most of us experience difficulty at some time remembering people's names.

Write the first letter of the person you want to remember on a piece of card. Sometime later, test yourself by looking at the card and trying to remember the name that begins with that first letter (Miller, 1975). Alternatively, run through the letters of the alphabet to see if any particular letter `feels' familiar to you as this may be the first letter of the name you wish to remember.

At the time of meeting a person, it is sometimes helpful to use 'visual imagery' to store the person's name in memory:

Some aspect that stands out or is unusual about a person's name should be pictured as a mental image. It might be that the person's name stands for a trade, like 'Mr Cooper' (barrel-maker). Alternatively, there might be something about that person that produces a picture in your mind (Yesavage, Rose & Bower, 1983); for example, to remember the name 'Carol' picture the person with a 'carrot' on her head, or with a 'pea' on top of 'Peter's' head.

One way to remember a list of details about a person (such as his or her name or age) is to make up a song or lyric that you can say to yourself every time you want to remember the information.

It is important to rehearse the lyric several times until you can remember it on a number of occasions without as much help from others (Gardner, 1977).

- **Names of objects**

This strategy works well for people with word-finding difficulty for everyday objects.

Get someone to tell you the word of an unfamiliar object when you use it in the way it is intended. In this way, every time you use the object you will know what it was called and the words for its function. You can also do this exercise by using pictures of objects and rehearsing the names over and over again. The more times you do this, the better (Karlsson et al, 1989; Thompson and Morgan, 1996).

- **Day, date and time**

People who have head a significant head injury are sometimes disorientated, especially during admission to an unfamiliar setting such as a rehabilitation unit and sometimes still later when they return home. People with dementia often experience disorientation.

Choose a time when you can regularly look at a calendar or a clock, for example, as soon as you get up in the morning. Write the date on a piece of card in large print and stick it on a wall in the kitchen (or somewhere you use regularly). It is helpful if someone else can ask you what time or day it is, so that you can rehearse these facts several times during the day (Godfrey & Knight, 1987).

- **What to buy**

'Self-statements' are sentences said to yourself. These can be invented for a particular problem.

For example: If you have difficulty remembering what to buy next, make a list of the items before you go shopping and choose a shop as a "safe haven" (for example, a clothes shop) that you will go into if you forget what to do next.
Then practice saying, 'I'll go into the clothes shop I know, whenever I forget the things I came for, and then I'll look at my shopping list' (Hussain, 1981). An alternative to a shop might be a

bench or statue or a prominent square in the town centre that you can return to in the event of forgetting items. These should act as a trigger or prompt for recall.

To remember a list of words, such as the items on the shopping list, picture each word with a familiar household object. For example, the word `potato' is pictured watching television and `sausages' are pictured taking a bath. When the words and pictures are well learned, go through the house in your mind picturing each piece of furniture and trying to remember the words (Robertson-Tchabo, Hausman & Arenberg, 1976).

A similar strategy involves pairing words (for example, items of a shopping list) to a familiar route or plan:

A string of onions is pictured hanging from the front door of your home, a bottle of milk on the doorstep, and half a dozen eggs on the inside door mat. When you are in the shop, simply think of your home in your mind. Each pictured item springs to mind as you walk your imagined route through your house.

More elaborate methods of using visual imagery and routes or stories are found elsewhere (see Buzan, 1989).

Teaching Memory Strategies to Others

There are numerous strategies that have been shown to be successful in alleviating some of the very distressing consequences of forgetting. Some methods are very elaborate; some are very simple to use. An essential part of using a strategy that focuses on `mental pictures' is the practice of producing a visual image. Some people find it easy to produce a picture of an item on request but others do not, just as some people dream in colour and others do not. Therefore, finding ways of producing mental pictures should be explored with the patient before a strategy can make use of this skill.

One way is to use *Progressive Muscle Relaxation* (PMR), such as the Jacobsonian abbreviated form. This method aims progressively to relax muscles beginning with the upper body (arms), then lower body (legs) and then shoulders, neck and face muscles (cheeks, forehead). Controlled breathing is taught at this stage and the patient is asked to think of a pleasurable scene such as lying on a beach in the sunshine or in the countryside. By practising PMR each day (about 15-20 minutes), the patient gradually acquires the skill of relaxation (in some cases re-learns how to relax) but, more importantly, learns how to produce a mental picture.

Learning how to relax is important since it is known that anxiety (Thompson, 1995) and depression (Thompson, 1992) can affect memory performance. Practising how to produce a visual image of different objects can then be carried out under these relaxed conditions in order to build-in this component into the memory strategy to be used. Many patients have benefited from this approach and it has been found to be useful when incorporated with a memory retraining programme for patients, for example in a memory clinic.

Amnesia can be very distressing and is commonplace among patients with head injuries and dementia. Different types of amnesia bring with them different problems, in terms of both definition and therapy. Understanding the processes involved in memory is paramount to knowing how best to help patients and a number of aids and strategies are available for use by the therapist.

Simple rehearsal has been found to be less useful for remembering information, although this does help the patient to 'know' or become familiar with information. Elaborative rehearsal, such as the peg system (Buzan, 1989), allows patients to remember items, but they may not 'know' the items since a reliance has been made on a sometimes abstract and meaningless strategy, albeit useful in recall.

Research has shown that patients learning how to help themselves by familiarising themselves with memory strategies have a better chance of improving their poor memory than simply by rehearsing items to be memorised (Richardson, 1992; Gardiner, Gawlik & Richardson-Klavehn, 1994), but careful assessment of the patient is essential to discern which strategies are most appropriate (Thompson, 1992; Wilson, 1992). For example, teaching a dense amnesiac patient the PQRST method has less value than strategies that strive to improve procedural memory. Examining everyday problems caused by memory deficits should also be considered in order to build up a total picture of the patient's problems for the therapist and which will be useful in establishing a retraining programme.

Finally, all strategies should be tailored to the individual needs and personality of the patient. For instance, you may prefer to imagine the scene of yourself sunbathing on a sandy beach in Cannes, whereas another person's mental picture might be basking on the pebbles in Bognor Regis (no preference implied!).

Figure 5.1   Using Word Association

Two couples were enjoying conversation on a park bench. One of the men said, "Bob, how was the memory clinic you went to the other day?"

"Amazing!", Bob replied. "They taught us the latest psychological techniques – one was visualisation, another one was association – it's made a big difference to my memory".

"That's great Bob! What was the name of the clinic?"

Bob went blank. He thought for a while but just couldn't remember. Then a smile broke across his face and he asked, "what do you call that flower with the long stem and thorns?"

"D'you mean a rose?"

"Yes, that's it!" He turned toward his wife... "Rose, what was the name of *that* clinic?"

Further Reading

Crook T.H. & Larrabee G.J. (1992) 'Normative data on a self-rating scale for evaluating memory in everyday life'. *Archives of Clinical*

Neuropsychology, 7, 41-51.

Gardiner J.I.M., Gawlik B. & Richardson-Klavehn A. (1994) 'Maintenance rehearsal affects knowing, not remembering; elaborative rehearsal affects remembering, not knowing'. *Psychonomic Bulletin and Review, 1 (1), 107-110.*

Richardson J.T.E. (1992) 'Imagery mnemonics and memory remediation'. *Neurology, 42,* 283-286.

Squires E.J., Hunkin N.M. & Parkin A.J. (1992) 'Memory notebook training in a case of severe amnesia: Generalising from paired associate learning to real life'. *Neuropsychological Rehabilitation,* 6 (1), 55-65.

Chapter 6

Advanced Memory Strategies

Before selecting a particular memory strategy that is suitable to your needs, it must be understood that not all techniques are suitable for everyone. Also, some techniques are best suited to only one modality, ie visual memory techniques will suit people who have difficulty in remembering things that they can see. Auditory techniques, based on hearing information, will be suitable for helping people remember things that they wish to remember hearing (eg the spoken word).

Hence, it is important to distinguish between visual and auditory memories. Different sites in the brain are responsible for different functions within the body. This is also true for memory functioning. This becomes clearer if we consider the different anatomical sites (within the brain) to which memory is attributed. For example, anterograde memory has been associated with the mammillary bodies (Kapur *et al.,* 1996b) (Fig. 2), whilst the temporal lobes (Fig. 3) are considered important for short-term memory (Lezak, 1995).

Other terms commonly used to describe memories are autobiographical and motor memory. Autobiographical memory is used to describe the ability to remember events and experiences from the past; motor memory involves remembering events and experiences from the actions required to perform them; eg remembering how to swim or how to ride a bicycle.

Key Points in Helping People to Learn Strategies

Repeated practice on memory tasks may bring some improvement but there is usually no generalisation to other tasks. It is therefore important to understand the techniques you are using and not just to rehearse them again and again. The following are some general principles that are used in retraining poor memory functioning:

- ensure that you are not distracted whilst learning your chosen technique.
- make sure that you understand the information you are reading.
- simplify the information you are reading and so reduce the

amount of information you have to remember.

- link what you have read to something else you have read or seen - link or "associate" it with other items.
- re-read the information for clarity and tackle the task often but a little at a time. It is better to understand something gradually than to try to understand it all at once and then forget it all.
- ensure that you try out the techniques in different situations. Try learning new techniques in relaxed situations and a variety of situations to make the task more interesting.

Berg, Koning-Haanstra and Deelman (1991) gave memory impaired patients a set of memory "rules" in an illustrated booklet which included the following:

1. Try to accept that a deficient memory cannot be cured.
2. Make more efficient use of your remaining memory capacities.
3. Use external aids where possible.
4. Pay more attention.
5. Spend more time.
6. Repeat.
7. Make associations.
8. Organise.
9. Link input and retrieval situations.

Other researchers have described particular methods of improving memory in different situations. For example, face-name associations, name-image associations, relating a memory to a place, rhymes, first letter cues (eg **R**ichard **O**f **Y**ork **G**ave **B**attle **I**n **V**ain = first letters of the colours of a rainbow: **R**ed, **O**range, **Y**ellow, **G**reen, **B**lue, **I**ndigo, **V**iolet), converting numbers to words, practical imitations (miming an action to remember a list of words or tasks). The following is a list of practical tips for adapting your environment and/or external aids:

- signposts
- reality orientation boards (day, date, etc.)
- coloured lines to the toilet
- differently coloured doors
- routines and prompts
- labels
- pictures to show contents of rooms, cupboards, drawers.
- diary
- notebook
- calendar
- alarms

- lists
- dictating machine
- portable tape recorder
- electronic organizer
- personal organiser

Remembering Complex Number Sequences

One of the hardest things people have to remember is numbers. Unfortunately, numbers appear in many different situations, such as house numbers, flat numbers, the time, how much you are paid, benefits, personal identification numbers for credit cards and cash machines, etc. Often there is no easy way to remember a string of numbers. However, visual imagery (imaging a scene or an object) is often a useful technique to use.

Alternatively, converting the numbers into letters allows you to remember them as a word instead of as number sequences. The following describes how you can do this. It is a complicated system but does work if you are able to dedicate some time to it.

Below is a series of letters beneath the numbers 0 to 9 which make up all the possible numbers you will wish to remember, simply by combination (ie 33 or 199, etc.). Only use vowels to create your "cueing" words - the vowels do not represent any of the numbers, only consonants are used. Also, only use the following letters to create words in the same way as the vowels: h, v, w, x, y.

0		1	2	3	4	5	6	7	8	9
zero/s/z		t/d	n	m	r/c	1		b/p	k	f	q/g/j

The first row beneath the numbers shows you how the "cueing" letters are derived from the number shapes. The second row shows you the letters you need to remember that represent each number. For example, to remember the number "43", you see that the letters "r" and "m" represent "4" and "3", respectively. Inserting a meaningless vowel (eg "a") in between gives you the cueing word "r a m" hence, to remember "43", remember "ram".

This technique sounds complicated but is actually quite easy to use once you have recognised the cueing letters. In time, you can use them to build up a complicated set of numbers to remember. It has the added advantage that you can stop and work out the representing letters from the number shapes if you happen to forget them.

In order to remember sequences of numbers, an alternative way is to remember a "matrix" of numbers (ie rows and columns of numbers).

s/z	t/d	n	m	r/c	1	b/p	k	F	q/g/j
_0	_1	_2	_3	_4	_5	_6	_7	_8	_9
10	11	12	13	14	15	16	17	18	19
20	21	22	23	24	25	26	27	28	29

Thus, to remember the row "4..14..24", remember the cueing letters: "r...... t..r...... n..r". Now insert some meaningless vowels and this makes:

r (oy)   tr (oy)   n (o)   r (oy)

or the non-sense saying, "roy troy no roy". Again, practicing the number shapes to form the cueing words enables you to build up an impressive set of number sequences. It doesn't matter how bizarre the saying is because no one else hears it and you are far more likely remembering something range strange.

In the end it is essential to select the techniques that you feel most comfortable using. They should be the ones that you find the easiest to use and also those that you understand the most easily.

Further Reading

Buzan T. (1989) *Master Your Memory*. London, David Charles.

Evans J.J. & Wilson B.A. (1992) 'A memory group for individuals with brain injury'. *Clinical rehabilitation, 6,* 75-81.

Glisky E.L., Schacter D.L. & Tulving E. (1986) 'Computer learning by memory impaired patients: Acquisition and retention of complex knowledge'. *Neuropsychologia,* 24 (3), 313-328.

Kennedy B.M. (1996) *Workbook for Memory Skills*. Florida, The Speech Bin Inc.

Parkin A.J. (1997) *Memory and Amnesia. An Introduction.* 2"[d] *Edn.* Oxford, Blackwell.

Swales M. & Johnson R. (1992) 'Patients with semantic memory loss: can they relearn lost concepts'? *Neuropsychological Rehabilitation, 2,* 295-306.

Chapter 7

Case Studies on Memory

Memory Clinics

Memory clinics have been established throughout the United Kingdom for assessing and rehabilitating out-patients who have specific memory impairment (Thompson *et al.,* 2001) and head injury. Guided by information and experience gained from a project which commenced in 1998, a new clinic was established, for one year, within the Older Persons Mental Health Services of the Sussex Weald and Downs NHS Trust.

This clinic attempted to establish the effects of Donepezil on visual memory in those patients with mild to moderate Alzheimer's Disease (Thompson *et al.,* 2001). The project was funded by Pfizer Pharmaceuticals and involved the recruitment of a liaison (CATE - Cognitive Assessment, Treatment and Evaluation) nurse to support the prescription of Aricept to selected patients, the evaluation of assessment tools and the psychosocial impact of treatment with Aricept. In addition, the Consultant Clinical Neuropsychologist assessed and monitored patients throughout the course of the study on neuropsyhological tests and clinical interviews.

Staffing Resource

It was agreed that the following staff was the minimum requirement:

- 0.2 whole time equivalent (WTE) Consultant Clinical Neuropsychologist
- 0.2 WTE Consultant in Old Age Psychiatry
- 0.2 WTE Senior Occupational Therapist
- 0.2 WTE Social Worker
- 0.2 WTE Community Psychiatric Nurses (Grade G x 3)
- 0.2 WTE Administration and clerical support.

Access to services such as Neurology and Speech and Language were co-ordinated as required, case by case.

Patient Inclusion Criteria

- Aged under 65 years
- Registered with a GP in the Chichester or Bognor Regis areas
- Symptoms of cognitive change or decline

Patient Exclusion Criteria

- Head injury

Referral Process

Directly to the co-ordinator of the memory clinic.

Publicity

An introductory newsletter was sent to all GPs, Consultants (from both the District General Hospital and psychiatric services) and Community Mental Health Teams in the Chichester and Bognor area two months before the first clinic. A second letter was then sent one month before the first clinic date.

Clinic Format

Appointments were allocated over a period of 4 - 5 visits to the clinic and were co-ordinated to link with screening processes and investigations. Appointments included a re-assessment component where performance and functioning were rated against earlier baseline measurements. Patients were always encouraged to attend with their partner or spouse, relative or close friend to assist with history taking and the assessment process.

Attendance at the Clinic

1. ***Consultant Psychiatrist or Specialist Registrar*** – Mini-Mental State Examination – MMSE (Folstein *et al.*, 1975); Addenbrooke's Cognitive Examination (Mathuranath *et al.*, 2000); Clinical Dementia Rating Scale (Hughes *et al.*, 1982); psychiatric examination, referral for testing (MRI/ CT/ fMRI etc), evaluation of all results and history taking, formulation of probable or actual diagnosis, commencement of treatment of cognitive or mood disorder as/if appropriate, review of interventions and

progress of disorder or response to treatment.

2. **Consultant Clinical Neuropsychologist** – Orientation questionnaire; Wechsler Memory Scale Revised (Wechsler, 1988) – a test of auditory verbal memory; Benton Visual Retention Test (Benton Sivan, 1992) – a test of visual memory and visuo-spatial skills; Wechsler Adult Intelligence Scale Revised (Wechsler, 1981) Digit Span sub-test – a test of immediate memory; Controlled Oral Word Association Test (Benton & Hamsher, 1983) – a verbal fluency test; Trail Making Test (Reitan, 1955; 1992) – to test motor co-ordination, information processing capacity and reaction times; educational package (Thompson, 2003) – advice and techniques from a memory book and information sheets.

3. **Senior Occupational Therapist** – Hospital Anxiety and Depression Scale (Zigmond & Snaith, 1983) – to assess anxiety and depression; Beck Depression Inventory (Beck *et al.*, 1996) – for a further in-depth assessment of depression; Disability Assessment for Dementia (Feldman *et al.*, 2001; Gélinas *et al.*, 1999) – for assessing problem-solving; Screen for Caregiver Burden – Modified (Gilleard, 1984); Severe Impairment Battery (Saxton *et al.*, 1993).

4. **Community Psychiatric Nurse (CPN)** – Home visit initial assessment and ongoing support throughout assessment period and subsequently, where appropriate. Also, Addenbrooke's Cognitive Examination and MMSE, if not previously completed.

5. **Social Worker** – Implementation of home care and support packages if appropriate, advice on social support services/finances/employment and care issues, child protection and liaison with other agencies.

The range of assessments undertaken within the service additionally included the Bristol Activities of Daily Living Scale (Bucks *et al.*, 1996), and the General Health Questionnaire (Goldberg & Williams, 1988). Furthermore, a full assessment of the patient's dietary patterns and intake, including alcohol, was undertaken. With the exception of neuropsychological testing undertaken by the Clinical Neuropsychologist, any of the assessments could be undertaken by any member of the team, dependent upon timing of visits and appointments and relationships established between professional and carer.

Evaluation and Monitoring

Clinic and referral data was collated by the co-ordinator and a clinical audit process conducted. A comparison with and impact on existing services was made and team opinion sought. The outcome and expectancies of the patients and those of the service providers was found to be positive and in favour of establishing an ongoing service.

The following table and charts (Table 7.1; Charts 7.1-7.4) show improvements in patients over the course of the study.

Table 7.1 Demographic Data (NART = National Adult Reading Test, an Estimate of Pre-morbid Intelligence or 'IQ')

	N	Age	NART Full IQ	NART Verbal	NART Perf
Male	6	72.5	88.5	88.67	90.50
		(6.69)	(7.23)	(6.92)	(6.66)
Female	10	74.4	101.60	100.60	101.90
		(5.66)	(10.47)	(9.77)	(9.52)
Total	16	73.69	96.69	96.13	97.63)
		(5.91)	(11.22)	(10.43)	(10.07)

Figure 7.1   Demographic Data (NART = National Adult Reading Test, an Estimate of Pre-morbid Intelligence or 'IQ')

Figure 7.2   Visual Memory Improvements

Figure 7.3   Verbal Memory Improvements

Dementia and Memory

Figure 7.4   Pre and Post Anxiety and Depression Scores

HADS Scales

PART III
Coping with Dementia

Chapter 8

How to Assess Dementia

Taking Histories

The family history can be of prime importance in a number of dementing illnesses, particularly in genetically inherited disorders such as Huntington's disease. The antecedent history may contain clues of great significance, and even slight head injury can lead to subdural haematoma (bleeding below the dural layer covering the brain), resulting in damage to nerve and brain tissue, and possibly subsequent infarcts or meningitis. It is also important to record fitting, faints and seizures, and neglect of diet may rule out some diagnoses or explain some symptoms (see Figures 8.1 and 8.2 for a guide to questioning the patient/carer). In all, a comprehensive account of the patient's lifestyle can considerably assist in an accurate diagnosis. In fact, very often a diagnosis of dementia is made after exclusion of other physical symptoms and organic origins. Special care should be taken to rule out the possibility of a differential diagnosis, for example between dementia and depression. Tools such as the Beck Depression Inventory (Beck & Steer, 1987) may be useful when used in conjunction with the clinical interview by a trained professional, for example a clinical psychologist.

Assessing Functions in People with Dementia

One problem that therapists and clinicians commonly face with people with memory problems, such as in dementia, is the classification of the severity of amnesia. Currently, there is no generally accepted classification except for a division in terms of performance on standardised tests of memory (Mayes, 1986), but this has limited value for real-life situations. Gordon (1987) has emphasised the importance of knowledge learnt in one setting and the patient's ability to generalise this knowledge to other settings. This seems to be a more useful measure of amnesic severity and it has uncontested usefulness in terms of therapeutic rehabilitation. Three levels of generalisation have been distinguished:

1. The results of training on a task should generalise from one session to the next, as well as to alternative forms of the training material.
2. Improvement should generalise to memory tests both similar to and different from the task which was trained.
3. Improvement should generalise from the particular task to everyday living.

Figure 8.1   Guidelines for a Structured Review

Name	Age	Date of birth
Address		Telephone
General practitioner Address		Telephone
Next of kin Address		Religion
Telephone		Marital status
Referred by Date referred Referral diagnosis		Date first seen
Medication		Laboratory results: Bloods Other (specify)

Detailed history

1   Psychological:

2   Social:

3   Physical (falls, head injuries, viruses, infections, etc.):

4   Onset:

5   Development:

6   Precipitating factors:

7   Relieving factors:

8 Help given to date:

9 Reasons for seeking help now:

10 Availability of support (and who?):

Impact of problem

1 Job:

2 Leisure/hobbies:

3 Relationships:

Own view of:

1 Problems:

2 Expectations of treatment:

3 Comments on past treatment:

Family history (age, occupation, amount and quality
of contact, health problems of family):

1 Father:

2 Mother:

3 Brothers and sisters:

4 Husband/wife/partner:

5 Children:

6 Relevant others:

7 Current family circumstances:

8 Home atmosphere:

Figure 8.2   Personal History

1	Infancy and childhood:
2	General health and nervous traits:
3	Personality:
4	School (age started, standard reached, attitude to school and school mates):
5	Work (age started, number of jobs, reasons for change, satisfaction level, ambitions):
6	Social life/network:

Intake of alcohol	tobacco	drugs
caffeine (coffee, tea, soft drinks)	Street drugs	

7	Leisure/hobbies:
8	Sexual history (menstrual history – how information gained; early sexual experience, distressing sexual experience, other):
9	Life events (achievements, bereavements):
10	Relevant topics not covered:

Clinician   *Date*

Source: Adapted from Thompson (1993b)

Glisky, Schacter and Tulving (1986) have warned that some patients with amnesia have great difficulty in level 3 generalisation. This can lead to 'hyperspecific learning', where recall can only take place if the conditions of learning are recreated precisely.

Environmental factors can influence assessment. Patients examined in a noisy setting, such as a room in a busy outpatient department or a part of the hospital that is particularly 'clinical' (with a clinical smell or plain walls) may perform less well (Thompson, 1995a). Sometimes the patient is very disorientated, and it may be necessary to establish the exact degree of disorientation the patient is experiencing; for example, the person may be unsure about the day or the month and year, or may not know their date of birth or where they are being assessed. A checklist is often useful to determine this knowledge (Figure 8.3), and can be used at frequent intervals to monitor the patient's level of orientation to their surroundings and circumstances. The Mini-Mental State Examination (Folstein, Folstein & McHugh, 1975) elaborates this type of questioning.

Figure 8.3   Orientation Questions

		Correct response	Patient's response	Tick/Cross
1	Patient's name:			
2	Day:			
3	Month:			
4	Date:			
5	Year:			
6	Place:			
7	Town:			
8	Prime Minister:			
9	Home address:			
10	Age:			
11	Date of birth:			
Total	Out of 11 (score ½ for items half-correct):			

Assessing Memory

There are a number of assessment tasks available to the trained therapist and clinician; for example, the Rivermead Behavioural Memory Test (Wilson, Cockburn & Baddeley, 1991) is useful in establishing the level of a patient's procedural memory functioning, but does not tell the clinician much about the patient's specific memory deficits, particularly in which modalities the deficits may be occurring (for example, visual or auditory).

More specific cognitive testing, using, for example, the Wechsler Memory Scale – Revised (WMS-R: Wechsler, 1981b), allows for identification of visual or auditory memory deficits, the patient's ability to learn new items ('new learning') and visuospatial deficits. If the patient has difficulty remembering particular words or people's faces, this deficit can be assessed using the Recognition Memory Test (RMT: Warrington, 1984). However, simple questioning of the patient about personal details, events and familiar routines also enables the therapist/clinician to gain a clinical impression of the patient's deficits and abilities.

It is also usually beneficial to interview the spouse, close relatives, carers or friends about the patient's past history, and the Autobiographical Memory Interview (AMI: Kopelman, Wilson & Baddeley, 1990) is particularly useful for this purpose.

Environmental factors can influence assessment. Patients examined in a noisy setting, such as a room in a busy out-patient department or a part of the hospital that is particularly 'clinical' (has a clinical smell or plain walls), may perform less well (Thompson, 1995). Particular brain-injury sites do cause specific and marked impairments (Damasio & Damasio, 1989; Hodges & McCarthy, 1993), including changes in the way a person displays his or her emotions, which may have a bearing on both the setting and method used by the therapist to assess the patient. The trauma of a brain injury can be so disorientating that it is little wonder that patients perform worse on admission than before discharge (Thompson, 1995).

The observation of patients in a number of functional settings and the recording of data to understand the everyday problems of brain-injured patients are invaluable to the assessment phase.

Assessing Cognitive Abilities

As part of the assessment process, the general practitioner or consultant may refer a suspected dementing patient to a rehabilitation team for an in-depth assessment. The membership of this team should include a clinical neuropsychologist, who will conduct a thorough investigation of the patient's abilities and deficits using a series of neuropsychological tests. The most common techniques are paper-and-pencil tests and requests to perform problem-solving or verbal ability tests, though assessment batteries vary according to what the clinician wishes to investigate. One commonly-used tool is the Wechsler Adult Intelligence Scale – Revised (WAIS–R: Wechsler, 1981a), which provides the clinician with an overall IQ, but more usefully, gives a profile of the patient's verbal and performance abilities on a variety of tests. Other tests, such as the Middlesex Elderly Assessment of Mental State (MEAMS: Golding, 1989), Kendrick Cognitive Tests for the Elderly (KCTE: Kendrick, 1985), Clifton Assessment Procedures for the Elderly (CAPE: Pattie & Gilleard, 1979) or the Dementia Rating Scale (DRS: Mattis, 1988a) are very useful screening tools for dementia, and can indicate the need for further testing in specific areas of deficits, such as memory for faces, recognition of everyday objects or arithmetic ability. (The reader is referred to specific texts on neuropsychology for more detail: for example, Lezak, 1983; Spreen & Strauss, 1991.)

Lishman (1987) warns that unless a full and comprehensive evaluation is made of a suspected dementing patient, labelling them with a primary dementing illness, for example, carries a hopeless prognosis. Care must be taken not only in carrying out tests but also in the interpretation of results. Hence, clinicians require a specific and detailed knowledge base to interpret results, even if the tests have been carried out by non-specialised, generic workers.

Monitoring Behaviour

The value of comprehensive inpatient evaluation has been shown by several surveys (Lishman, 1987). Often, the ability to monitor a patient closely is enhanced in an inpatient setting; however, these settings can be too clinical and unrepresentative of the patient's true home setting. Therefore, a compromise must be made, where the patient can be monitored either in both settings or by a professional visiting the patient at home.

A number of methods for observing patients can be considered. For example, the patient may be observed discretely by another sitting in the corner of a room. Each time an 'event' or observable behaviour occurs, the behaviour (B) is recorded, together with a brief description of what was happening just prior to that event (A – antecedent) and the consequence (C). In this way, an A-B-C chart may be completed, which can help discern any patterns of behaviour in the client, or can help discover the reasons for a particular piece of repeated (and possibly distressing/unsociable) behaviour (see Figure 8.4).

Figure 8.4   The A-B-C Chart

A = Antecedent	B = Behaviour	C = Consequence
(What was happening, and where was the person before the behavious was observed?)	*(Describe the actual behaviour observed.)*	*(What happened, and where, as a consequence of the behaviour?)*
Simon entered the ward; Natalie was lying on her bed sleeping.	Natalie leapt up and screamed.	Three nurses rushed to Natalie's bedside to see what was happening.
David was sitting in the day room.	David vomited violently on the floor.	A nurse attended to David and cleaned up the vomit.

Alternatively, a more detailed record may be completed, such as a time sampling record. In this case, at the end of every minute for a period of 30 minutes, for example, all observable behaviour is observed and recorded. In this instance, it is helpful to use the first few minutes just to record the sort of behaviour being presented

Figure 8.5 Interval Sampling Record

Client:
DOB:
Time Period:

Date:
Clinician:
Where Recorded:

Time interval (mins)	Sits quietly still	Look towards others (O) object (OJ)/ downwards (D)	Leaves seat	Stereotyped movements: rocks in chair; both hands held together resting on lap	Starts to strip	Teeth grinding	Throws object	Frowns (F) or smiles (S)	Stretches one arm out to object	Interaction by staff (specify)	Other behaviour (specify) e.g. feeding; moves cushion behind self
1											
2											
3											
4											
5											
6											
7											
8											
9											
10											
11											
12											
13											
14											
15											
16											
17											
18											
19											
20											
21											
22											
23											
24											
25											
26											
27											
28											
29											
30											

in order to draw up column headings of 'behaviours' which can be ticked later as they are observed (see Fig 8.5). A third type of record is an event sampling record where simply the time when an event is first observed is noted and then the time when it finishes (or when it is stopped by someone else). It is useful to add a 'comments' section for clarification when analysing the data later on (Figure 8.6).

Figure 8.6	**Event Sampling Record**	
Event 1:	Dave pushes Neal out of the way.	
Time:	Start:	10:45:07 a.m.
	Stop:	10:45:37 a.m.
Comment:	Behaviour observed for 30 seconds before staff intervened.	
Event 2:	Dave taps table with fists repeatedly.	
Time:	Start:	11:05:11 a.m.
	Stop:	11:10:11 a.m.
Comment:	Dave stopped spontaneously.	
Event 3:	Dave says he is sorry to Neal.	
Time:	Start:	12:16:02 p.m.
	Stop:	12:16:32 p.m.
Comment:	Dave does not look at Neal when he says sorry.	
Event 4:	Dave puts his sock on over his shoe.	
Time:	Start:	14:03:00 p.m.
	Stop:	14:08:01 p.m.
Comment:	Bev and Paul show him that he is already wearing a sock and shoe.	

Sometimes the professional wishes to record only one particular type of behaviour during an observation; for example, the patient may have a habit of collecting items of food and storing them in their sleeve and forgetting they have put them there afterwards. In this case, the single behaviour may occur before or after, for example, visiting the toilet and then the kitchen. A delayed (or time lag) or event lag record may be used where the time is recorded at the start and finish of the target behaviour (which may be lagging behind another different behaviour being observed – hence 'event or time lag'). The simplest of all recording, however, is a description of the behaviour and events over an allotted period of time. This is usually more reliable than a diary completed from memory or a verbatim account of events after they have happened. Whether by a professional (for example, a community occupational therapist, clinical psychologist, nurse, social worker or carer) or a relative or friend, all of these types of records can be completed following some explanation of the reason and the importance for their completion.

Methodological Considerations and Applicability of Tests

Besides diagnostic uncertainty, there are a number of methodological issues that complicate the understanding of dementia, depression and their interaction. One of these is the fact that the course of many dementias covers a relatively long time span. Longitudinal studies are therefore favoured but these bring with them the problems of funding and resources, and natural attrition of subjects. There are also problems in gaining consent for participation in research and permission from next of kin in the case of post-mortem analysis (see Hagberg & Gustafson, 1985).

Applicability of test material that is already available and standardised is also an important consideration; this raises not only the question of transferability of norms to other client groups (for example, people with learning disabilities), but also of whether adapted or modified tests become invalid following alterations to the format or content of the tests. In particular, the Wechsler Adult Intelligence Scale (WAIS: Wechsler, 1955) and WAIS-R (Wechsler, 1981a), have been the focus of attention (for example, Moulin, 1980; Jones, 1987; Atkinson, 1991a).

The 11 sub-tests of the WAIS-R provide data on a 'general intelligence' (g) factor, as well as two or three factorially-derived group dimensions (Wechsler, 1981a). In addition, each sub-test measures certain 'specific' or 'unique' abilities: capacities that are not assessed by the other subscales (Leckliter, Matarazzo & Silverstein, 1986). Central to the diagnostic endeavour is a need to distinguish variation between sub-tests that can be attributed to measurement error, and variation that reflects a true difference in underlying abilities (Atkinson, 1991a). McNemar (1957) published a table of reliabilities, standard deviations and standard errors of measurement of *difference scores* for the WAIS. These statistics enable the clinician to determine the extent to which difference scores can be attributed to measurement error, and the extent to which they reflect true differences across ability levels. Piedmont, Sokolove and Fleming (1989) published figures for interpreting WAIS-R difference scores based on a sample of 229 psychiatric patients (and recommended fuller exploration of the WAIS-R with more homogeneous clinical samples).

Atkinson (1991b) produced a similar table describing the properties of sub-test score differences for the WAIS-R standardisation sample. He argued that calculations used by McNemar (1957) and Piedmont, Sokolove and Fleming (1989) were technically incorrect for generalising beyond their samples, since their standard error of measurement (which he claimed was purely descriptive in nature) provided an inflated estimate of the population parameter (for a full explanation of standard errors and difference scores, see Lord & Novick, 1968; Dudek, 1979). Atkinson's (1991a) data, based on a sample of 290 individuals with 'developmental delay', provides a better estimate, and enables a modification to be made to raw sub-test scores, obtained by using the WAIS-R, in order to test significant differences between individual test items. While potentially a very useful tool, Atkinson (1991a) warns that his sample is not presented as 'normative' for the learning disability population; nevertheless, he suggests the tables provide a 'tentative empirical yardstick'. However, this leaves clinicians and researchers with limited and non-generalisable norms to compare across people, for example, with a range of learning disabilities.

Some Conclusions about Assessment

Assessing patients with a suspected diagnosis of dementia is largely dependent upon:

1. who the asseesssor is (carer, relative, professional, etc);
2. what the assessor wishes to find out;
3. why this information is required.

Assessments are as varied as the knowledge base of each assessor; for example, a clinical neuropsychologist may wish to assess the extent to which dementia has affected the individual in terms of cognitive abilities (memory, concentration), personality (depression, changes in mood and attitude) and perception. There may be some shared areas of assessment with the occupational therapist, who will also wish to know how the individual's cognitive abilities have been affected, but perhaps with particular reference to how the individual performed previously in their job, home surroundings or interactions with family and friends. Adaptation of equipment and furniture may be considered necessary, together with the need for home help and carers.

As a team, findings of an assessment should be shared, if only to avoid duplication of assessment measures, but more importantly, to share opinions and experience and to co-ordinate a consistent and unitary approach to the care of the patient.

'Assessment' therefore means different things to different people, but answers to the three questions posed above should be along the following lines:

Q1   Who is the assessor?
A1   Occupational therapist.
Q2   What do you wish to find out about the individual?
A2   How the individual used to function in his/her home environment, both functionally and cognitively (level of independence, memory and sociability).
Q3   Why is this information needed?
A3   To feed back to the Rehabilitation Team and to provide relatives and carers with advice about management of the patient. Also, to establish realistic expectations of the patient.

Once the 'philosophy' is right for conducting the assessment, then hopefully, the findings will be meaningful and useful to the assessor. There is little worse than to conduct an assessment without either knowing why you are doing it or knowing why you are using a particular assessment tool. Consultation with others involved in the care of the dementing patient is therefore of paramount importance.

Summary of Functions that should be Assessed

The following is a non-exhaustive, 'rapid' checklist of areas and functions relevant to the patient that should be assessed. Theses will depend upon the assessor and the reasons for the assessment, as discussed above:

1   *Social and Psychiatric (all disciplines?)*

•   Explore the home environment.
•   Investigate family support.
•   Find out who is available/willing to offer long-term help.
•   Evidence of dementia in the family? (How was it dealt with?).
•   Obtain a detailed family history.

2 *Medical*

Refer patient for neuro-imaging (brain scan): MRI, CT or Single Photon Emission Tomography (SPECT). *Functional* MRI scans and SPECT scans are also available. These may help exclude other organic abnormalities in the brain structure or vascular causes, such as stroke.

- Take blood tests.
- Check the cardiovascular system.
- Confirm the diagnosis.
- Maintain good general health.

3 *Nursing*

- Maintain current activities, where possible.
- Maintain good general health.
- Prevent/treat bed sores.
- Prevent further illness/treat further illness.
- Establish a set daily routine for the patient.
-

4 *Neuropsychological Assessment*

- Memory;
- Perception;
- Language;
- Executive functions (e.g., ability to plan and organise);
- Ability to understand;
- Emotional adjustment/awareness of disability;
- Changes in personality;
- Current and premorbid intelligence.

5 *Speech and Language*

- Conversation;
- Written tasks;
- Higher language ability;
- Requests;
- Commands.

6 *Occupational Therapy*

- Everyday living skills;
- Mobility;

- Emotional adjustment to disability;
- Awareness of disability;
- Family support;
- Adaptations;
- Seating and positioning (including chairs, wheelchairs, beds).
-

7 *Physiotherapy*

- Exercise and mobility;
- Cardiovascular and muscular activity;
- Positioning (including chairs, wheelchairs, beds);
- Handling.
-

8 *Social Work*

- Investigate links/help from relatives, friends, carers;
- Benefits (financial aid);
- Grants (for equipment, adaptations);
- Housing requirements, residential homes, hostels;
- Access to community resources;
- Willingness to use facilities/willingness to co-operate.

Ideally, a report should be sought from each professional discipline, including the family doctor, who may have known the patient for several years. Discussion and an exchange of ideas is usually beneficial, and should, where possible, also include the carer, friend or relative and the patient, especially in any decisions that are made about the patient.

Further Reading

Baddeley, A.D., Wilson, B.A. & Watts, F. (1995), *Handbook of Memory Disorders*, Chichester: John Wiley.

Haycox, J. (1984), 'A simple reliable clinical behavioral scale for assessing demented patients', *Journal of Clinical Psychiatry*, **45**: 23–4.

Kapur, N. (1994), *Memory Disorders in Clinical Practice*, Hove: Lawrence Erlbaum.

Lezak, M.D. (1983), *Neuropsychological Assessment*, (2nd edn), New York: Oxford University Press.

Mattis, S. (1988b), 'Mental status examination for organic mental syndrome in the elderly patient', in Bellak, L. & Karasu, T. (eds), *Geriatric Psychiatry: A Handbook for Psychiatrists and Primary Care*

Physicians, New York: Grune & Stratton.

McCue, M., Rogers, J.C. & Goldstein, G. (1990), 'Relationships between neuropsychological and functional assessment in elderly neuropsychiatric patients', *Rehabilitation Psychology*, **35**: 91–5.

Nussbaum, P.D., Goreczny, A. & Haddad, L. (1995), 'Cognitive correlates of functional capacity in elderly depressed versus patients with probable Alzheimer's disease', *Neuropsychological Rehabilitation*, **5**, 4: 333–40.

Spreen, O. & Strauss, E. (1991), *A Compendium of Neuropsychological Tests: Administration, Norms and Commentary*, New York: Oxford University Press.

Tout, K. (1993), *Elderly Care: A World Perspective*, London: Chapman & Hall.

Tulving, E. (1983), *Elements of Episodic Memory*, New York: Oxford University Press.

Yesavage, J.A., Brink, T.L., Rose, T.L., Lum, D., et al. (1983), 'Development and screening of a geriatric depression rating scale: A preliminary report', *Journal of Psychiatric Research*, **7**: 37–49.

Chapter 9

How to Cope with Dementia

Medical Treatment of Dementia

Maintaining good physical health is important if the patient's deterioration is to be slowed. Ensuring adequate nutrition and hydration, with vitamin minerals and iron supplements, if necessary, is important to the overall health of the patient, and allows the clinician or carer to make the best use of residual functions. Lishman (1987) advises directing particular attention to the lungs and urinary tract, where infections, especially in bed-rested patients, can be a considerable problem if not avoided or managed carefully early on.

Urinary tract infections in particular can lead to confusion and disorientation. Congestive cardiac failure, cardiac arrhythmia and hypertension should be managed with special care. Careful monitoring of drug toxicity and control of anticoagulants is especially important for patients with multi-infarct dementia, and adequate physical exercise should be encouraged, whether at home or by visiting local physiotherapy services.

Sometimes it is appropriate to prescribe psychotropic medication: for example, anxiolytics to help reduce agitation or anxiety. Antidepressants can also be helpful where the patient is known to be depressed, but where possible, the patient should be offered counselling and psychological interventions, such as cognitive behavioural therapy for depression, which can be provided by the clinical psychology service, increasingly based at medical centres, general practitioner practices, health clinics or local hospitals.

Phenothiazines can sometimes transform the problems of management in a distressed or restless patient; they have benefits over barbiturates, which tend to aggravate confusion in older patients. A number of other drugs have been tried with dementing patients: for example, ribonucleic acid (Cameron & Solyom, 1961), magnesium pemoline (Cameron, 1967), pentylenetetrazol (Prien, 1973), pipradol (Turek et al., 1969), procaine and novocaine injections, pyrithoxin, cytidine, uridine and meclofenoxate (Villa & Ciompi, 1968) and hyperoxygenation (Jacobs et al., 1969; Edwards & Hart, 1974; Thompson et al., 1976).

Unfortunately, drug trials attempting to rectify the cholinergic effects in Alzheimer's disease patients have not been very successful (Corkin et al., 1982), while medical intervention for Parkinson's disease, Huntington's disease and multiple sclerosis have seen some success mainly in reducing some of the extrapyramidal system abnormalities. Pallidectomy and thalamotomy have also been tried in order to control abnormal motor movements. Heathfield (1967) concluded that younger patients with minimal mental changes, good insight and severe chorea (as in Huntington's chorea) had better chances of improvement with these surgical interventions, whereas they have tended to aggravate dementia, especially in older patients.

Amantadine has been used in the management of Creutzfeldt-Jakob disease, though the research findings must be interpreted with some caution. Braham (1971) reported marked improvement in a particular patient he studied, although the patient suffered a relapse, and Sanders and Dunn (1973) reported two successes, although in one patient the diagnosis was not proven. These authors have suggested that a metabolic rather than an antiviral action of the drug was involved in these patients, especially since in one patient the response appeared to be dose-related. Sanders (1979) has reported a further example of considerable temporary improvement in a 56-year-old man, while Ratcliffe et al. (1975) and Kovanen, Haltia and Cantell (1980) have found no benefit. Other drugs have also been tried, such as interferon (used in the management of multiple sclerosis), but with little or no success.

Among the many neurological and neurochemical abnormalities that develop in Alzheimer's disease are cell loss and malfunctioning of cholinergic neurones. Actylcholine is an important neurotransmitter associated with memory. Alterations in the enzyme ssystems involved in cholinergic function, ie choline acetyl transferase (Chat) and acetyl choline esterase (AchE) together with loss of cholinergic neurones are amongst the most consistent finings in Alzheimer's disease (Sutherland et al., 1995).

Aricept (donepezil Hydrochloride, E2020), an acetylcholineesterase inhibitor, acts to increase the availablity of acetylcholine within the synapses of neurones which remain intact in the brains of individuals with Alzheimer's disease (Weinstock, 1999) (Fig 6.1). This offers the possibility of improved neuronal function.

The effects of medication on visual memory deficits and visuo-spatial impairment in Alzheimer's disease have not been widely documented until recently (Thompson, MacDonald and Coates, 2001). It is argued that Aricept has been shown to have modest benefits though with small but significant improvements in cognitive functioning with 5 or 10 mg per day doses (Bryson & Benfield, 1997). In the Thompson et al, 2001 study, visual memory and visuo-spatial skills, and auditory verbal memory scores improved following a course of Aricept. These findings were extremely encouraging and are consistent with past indicators of improved cognitive functioning following Aricept prescription. The findings were thought to be unique at the time and research into the visual memory deficits and Alzheimer's disease is ongoing particulary with other "anti-dementia" drugs such as Reminyl (Galantamine Hydrobromide), Exelon (Rivastigmine Tartrate) and Ebixa (Memantine).

Offering Patients a Whole Package of Care

It is important to consider the specific needs of the person with dementia. While some may require considerable help with memory functioning, others may require help with coming to terms with the diagnosis in the first instance. Support is often also needed for carers and relatives, who sometimes feel a form of bereavement, especially if they feel that they have 'lost' the person they used to know because their personality or behaviour has changed.

Actual grief may also be experienced as friends of older people die or the patient with dementia dies leaving a bereaved partner. Specific help may be on offer in a number of ways; either direct support from professionals trained in bereavement counselling, clinical psychologists, nurse specialists and social workers, or voluntary organisations. Other help may be sought from *The Bereavement and Loss Training Manual* (Goodall, Drage & Bell, 1995), or from formal workshops that provide training for several different groups of professionals, for example, 'Working with Older People' (Murphy & Langley, 1995). The rehabilitation setting, whether a day centre or inpatient facility, should be able to provide the patient with a range of specifically-trained professionals or contacts whereby the patient (or their carer) may seek support or help. In areas where this is not the case, the general practitioner should be approached in the first instance for guidance.

Reality Orientation

Sometimes there is a blurring of boundaries between what is reality orientation and what is memory re-training. After all, we all rely on our memories to be orientated to our environment. However, orientation also depends upon environmental cueing; some of these cues can be very subtle, such as hearing familiar noises (for example, birds singing signifying early morning, or a car starting in the street). Some cues may be the date on the top of a newspaper or consulting a wristwatch for the correct time.

Reality orientation is important, especially to older, confused people, and can be maintained relatively simply by using large, clear calendars, and clocks with a large face. Bringing patients up-to-date with current affairs can be achieved through discussion groups or by individual questioning, and sometimes aids for reminiscence are useful, either for prompting memory or for orientation. Examples of such aids include radio theme tunes from the 1940s and 1950s, photographs of particular entertainers and personalities from various eras, and 'treasured' memories of important events (whether generally historical or of personal significance to the patient).

Scrapbooks of such items provide both involvement and important reminiscence for dementing patients, and should not be dismissed because of their apparent simplicity or banality. Collecting together items to produce a 'life story' for the patient can be rewarding, both for the patient and their partner, and can serve as reminiscence therapy and prompts for memory functioning. Whenever such approaches are explored, it is also useful to explore the family mechanisms for support that are currently in place. Identifying which family members wish to help in therapy can be invaluable, to both patient and carer, providing general support and enhancing welfare.

Further Reading

Baddeley, A.D. (1996), *Human Memory* (revised edn), Hove: Psychology Press.

Bennett, G. & Kingston, P. (1993), *Elder Abuse: Concepts, Theories and Interventions*, London: Chapman & Hall.

Burnside, I. (1990), 'Reminiscence research: An independent nursing intervention', *Issues in Mental Health Nursing*, **11**, 1: 33–8.

Kovach, C.R. (1990), 'Promise and problems in reminiscence research', *Journal of Gerontology*, **16**, 4: 10–14.

Miller, E. (1975), 'Impaired recall and memory disturbance', *British Journal of Social & Clinical Psychology*, **14**: 73–9.

Penson, J. (1990), *Bereavement: A Guide for Nurses*, London: Chapman & Hall.

Yesavage, J.A., Rose, T.L. & Bower, G.H. (1983), 'Interactive imagery and affective judgements improve face-name learning', *Journal of Gerontology*, **38**, 2: 198–203.

Chapter 10

How to Manage Dementia

Psychological and Social Management of Dementia

The term 'management' should be distinguished from 'treatment' in the context of this book: the former seeks to maintain current medical and psychological states in the patient, while the latter infers an approach or intervention, rather than a coping strategy. The two terms probably blend together when considering the longer-term care of a person with dementia, in that 'treatment' often becomes a long-term approach, which in turn 'manages' the condition. However, for the purposes of this book, 'management' will refer to maintenance of the person's overall welfare and stability, both medically and psychologically. Sometimes, the term 'coping' is preferred and subsumes both 'management' and 'treatment'.

Considerable support for both patient and carer (whether a relative or a paid professional) is often needed. The social work service can assist with advice regarding benefits and housing, but often they can also provide expertise in counselling and supporting people faced with the many sudden changes associated with dementia. Attendance at day centres, help with using community resources, 'meals on wheels' and contact with voluntary organisations is usually welcomed by carers of dementing patients who may feel socially isolated, helpless and otherwise unsupported.

The family of the dementing person should also be explored for social and psychological support. Macmillan (1960) has discussed the common progression seen in the families of older demented patients, whereby responsibility is at first willingly accepted but later this is seen to become an increasing burden and is less accepted by family members. The clinical psychologist can also provide help in this respect by addressing the frequently emerging feelings of shame, and even denial of the family member having dementia. Fear about the course of the disease is evidenced not only by patients themselves but also by family members, who may also face a similar fate when they are older. Support from professionals is essential, especially at the time when admission of the dementing patient to hospital is required, or in the latter stages of the disease when the family can no longer care for the patient.

It is especially important to maintain self-esteem in patients with dementia. Kennedy (1959) has described how dementing patients commonly develop a sense of ill-formulated inferiority. Reassurance and empathy are important ingredients in any psychological intervention for these patients.

Several authors have emphasised the need to make the optimal use of residual functions, and to keep the patient correctly orientated in time, space and person in order to achieve this aim. Cosin et al. (1958) were able to demonstrate the effectiveness of simple occupational and social activities in improving, at least in the short term, the general level of behaviour of older patients with dementia. Domestic activities, particularly those involving cooperation with others, produced the most noticeable stimulation and satisfaction. Bower (1967) has also shown how the effects of an enriched environment can slow down or even reverse obvious evidence of the dementing process over a discrete time period. Environmental stimulation, such as multi-sensory rooms (Thompson & Martin, 1994) and 'Snoezelen' (Hulsegge & Verheul, 1987; Hutchinson, 1991; Long & Haig, 1992), has been shown to be therapeutic for older people (Willcocks, 1994), as well as for people with learning disabilities (Haggar & Hutchinson, 1991; Thompson & Martin, 1993; 1994). Others have claimed successes in modifying challenging behaviour resulting from dementia with token economy regimes (Miller, 1977; Woods & Britton, 1977).

What these studies tell us is that any approach should be tailored to the individual needs of the patient, and that there may be different expectations between patients, largely dependent on personality and the extent of residual functions. Above all, the patient should be encouraged to lead as normal a life as possible, with the necessary prompts and routines put in place to maximise, as far as possible, opportunities to maintain their independence.

Using Progressive Muscle Relaxation

Progressive Muscle Relaxation (PMR) exercises may be helpful in conjunction with chosen memory strategies in order to teach the individual to become more relaxed and therefore, more prepared to learn new information. It is well known that anxiety and depression, and hypertension, all impede the ability to remember information by virtue of the fact that a tense individual is less likely to be able to remember information or carry out even well-learned tasks.

PMR exercises are intended to relax the individual and are not necessarily intended to improve sleeping patterns. Therefore, these exercises should be carried out at a regular time each week, preferably daily, but several hours before bed time. They are an abbreviated version of the Jacobsonian PMR which usually takes 1.5 to 2 hours to carry out. This version should only take approximately 20 minutes.

If you prefer, you may talk these instructions into a portable tape recorder or dictating machine so that they can be played back at your leisure. However, it is advisable to read through the instructions first so that you are familiar with them and also to speak calmly and clearly into the tape recorder. (The Author grants permission for personal use within copyright.)

The following instructions are written below in the style of someone reading them out loud. You may wish to adapt them according to your needs.

1. Use a comfortable chair in a quiet room where you know that you are not going to be disturbed for 20 minutes.
2. Make yourself comfortable in the chair and close your eyes.
3. Try and shut out all other noises around you and listen to the instructions. In a moment I am going to ask you to raise your arms above your head, to point your fingers towards the ceiling and to stretch your arms, tightening the muscles in your arms as much as possible. I am going to ask you to hold then there until the count of five.
4. Right, raise both your arms above your head for five. Right, raise both your arms above your head, point your fingers towards the ceiling and hold them there for the count of five. One Two Three Four Five.
5. Let your arms go now; relax your arms. Return your arms back to your lap. Notice the difference in the muscles in your arms. Notice how relaxed they are now.
6. In a moment I am going to ask you to stretch both your legs out in front of you and to point your toes towards the opposite wall.
7. Right, raise both your legs slightly above the floor, stretch your legs. Tighten the muscles in your legs and point your toes towards the opposite wall. Hold them there for the count of five. One Two Three Four Five.
8. Let your legs drop to the floor now. Notice the floor pushing up against your feet. Your legs are now relaxed. The muscles in your legs are relaxed. Notice how relaxed your legs are now. Notice how heavy they are now. In a moment I am going to ask

you to put some extra tension in the muscles in your neck and shoulders and in your face.

9. Move your chin towards your chest. Hunch your shoulders so that they are tight and wrinkle your face. Pull a funny face and hold it all there for the count of five. One Two Three Four Five.

10. Let it all go now. Just relax. Let the muscles in your face relax. Have a blank expression now and let your shoulders just relax. Notice how heavy your neck and shoulders are now. Notice how relaxed and heavy the muscles are in your shoulders and in your neck.

11. In a moment I am going to ask you to do all three exercises at once. I am going to ask you to raise both your arms above your head, to point your fingers towards the ceiling, to raise both your legs slightly above the floor, to point your toes towards the opposite wall. I am going to ask you to hunch your shoulders and to scrunch your face and put your chin down to meet your chest and to hold it all there until the count of five.

12. Right, raise both your arms above your head, pointing your fingers towards the ceiling. Raise your legs stretched out, slightly above the floor, pointing your toes towards the opposite wall and scrunch up your face, hunch your shoulders and bring your chin down to meet your chest. Hold it all there until the count of five. One Two Three Four Five.

13. Right, let it all go now. Let your arms just rest gently on your lap. Let the muscles just become heavy and relaxed. Let your legs go. Feel the floor pushing against your feet and let your shoulders return, feeling heavy and relaxed. Make sure you have a blank expression on your face. Just sitting there calm and relaxed. Try and force out all the tension and tightness in your muscles. Force out that energy and just to sit there quietly and relaxed. 14. Notice how heavy your arms and your legs and your shoulders now feel.

14. I want you to think about your breathing now. Try and breathe out slightly more than you breathe in.

15. Breathe quietly and slowly.

16. Try to picture a pleasant scene such as lying on a beach in the sunshine or lying relaxed in the countryside.

17. Take a few minutes to enjoy your scene. Lying there quiet and relaxed.

18. In a moment, I want you to think about beginning to open your eyes. When I count backwards from five, I want you to start to open your eyes. Five Four Three Two One. Okay, start to open your eyes now. Open your eyes now.

These exercises may be repeated if necessary but it is important to give these instructions clearly and slowly and in a language that the individual understands. These instructions are provided only as a guide and do not have to be read out exactly. However, it is important for the whole series of exercises to be carried out in a quiet, and preferably, slow manner.

'Memory' often uses visual imagery, so try to practice picturing a pleasant scene whilst relaxing.

Further Reading

Gibson, H.B. (1991), *The Emotional and Sexual Lives of Older People*, London: Chapman & Hall.

Green, J.B. (1991), *Dealing with Death: Practices and Procedures*, London: Chapman & Hall.

Long, A.P. & Haig, L. (1992), 'How do clients benefit from Snoezelen? An exploratory study', *British Journal of Occupational Therapy*, **55**, 3: 103–6.

Matson N & Williams C *(1983) Coping with Memory Difficulties.* Exeter, Royal Devon and Exeter Hospital.

Willcocks, S. (1994), 'Snoezelen in elderly care' (conference report)', *British Journal of Occupational Therapy*, **57**, 6: 242.

Wilson, B.A. & Moffat, N. (1992), *Clinical Management of Behavioural Problems*, London: Chapman & Hall.

Chapter 11
Case Studies on Dementia

Clinical Trials

Perhaps the most researched area of all the dementias is that of Alzheimer's disease. As well as being one of the most prevalent conditions, it has also received considerable interest from a number of pharmaceutical companies at various times. However, this area of research has often come under scrutiny and has been criticised (for example, Swash et al., 1991).

Various researchers and working parties (for example, the Medical Research Council, 1987) have looked at the way research into dementia has been conducted in the past. It is of fundamental importance that even initial clinical trials of new treatments should be scientifically rigorous (Leber, 1986); inadequately-planned pilot trials may make it difficult or impossible to conduct a full and adequate trial at a later date (Swash et al., 1991).

Since no specific diagnostic test is available, the diagnosis of Alzheimer's disease remains a matter of clinical decision-making. However, this problem has been addressed by McKhann, Drachman and Folstein (1984) and by a working party (Tierney, Fisher & Lewis, 1988) who have suggested criteria for definite, probable and possible Alzheimer's disease. Similar criteria have been validated by clinical and pathological studies, yielding a sensitivity of 80 per cent and a specificity of 78 per cent (Wade, Mirsen & Hachinski, 1987).

Alzheimer's disease and cerebral vascular disease may coexist, as they are both common in older people (Rosen, Terry & Fuld, 1980). As Swash et al. (1991) comment, patients with this combination of disorders are generally not suitable for research studies of Alzheimer's disease itself; for research studies generally, the clinical diagnosis should be supported by quantitative assessments of the abnormality in intellectual function, for example by application of the Mini-Mental State Examination (Folstein, Folstein & McHugh, 1975), the Blessed Dementia Scale (Blessed, Tomlinson & Roth, 1968), the Cambridge Cognitive Examination (Roth, Tym & Mountjoy, 1986), the Geriatric Mental State Test (Folstein, Anthony & Parhad, 1985; Hughes, Berg

& Danziger, 1982), or by neuropsychological (Huppert & Tym, 1986) and other tests, for example, the National Adult Reading Test (Nelson & Willison, 1991), as a measure of premorbid intellect (Hart, 1988).

Scales of functional improvement, however, may include behavioural (Haycox, 1984) and cognitive tests (Huppert & Tym, 1986), assessments of the quality of life achievable by the patient, and scales of activities of daily living and functional competence (Lawton & Brody, 1969; Linn & Linn, 1983; Kuriansky, 1976). Secondary effects related to the amount of attention given by the researchers can be obviated by the use of a randomised placebo treat-ment arm (Swash et al., 1991), and depressive features may similarly be controlled (Agbayewa et al., 1991; Henderson & Huppert, 1985; Nussbaum, Goreczny & Haddad, 1995).

Working Memory in Alzheimer's Disease

In 1986, Baddeley et al. explored the hypothesis that patients suffering from dementia of the Alzheimer's type are particularly impaired in the functioning of the central executive component of working memory. Impaired memory is one of the earliest and most characteristic symptoms of Alzheimer's disease (Wilcock et al., 1989), a symptom that particularly reveals itself in complaints of lapses of memory in everyday life (Baddeley et al., 1991).

Many studies of short-term memory in Alzheimer's disease have attempted to establish how such memory deficits fit into the working memory model of Baddeley (1986, 1992). The model includes a central executive system (CES), which functions to co-ordinate and schedule different mental operations, including the processing and immediate storage of information. The CES controls the functioning of the separate storage mechanisms, the main ones being the phonological or articulatory loop system (ALS) and the visuospatial sketchpad (VSSP). The ALS acts as a repository for verbally-encoded items combined with a rehearsal mechanism, which recycles verbal material to refresh the memory trace, while the VSSP retains visuospatial material in short-term memory (Figure 11.1).

Figure 11.1 Schematic based on Baddeley's (1992) Working Memory Model

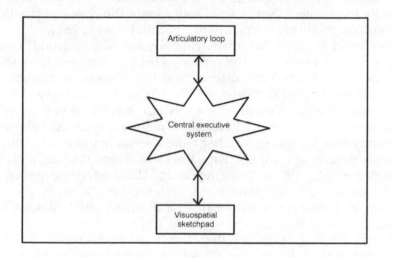

As Morris (1994a) explains, the CES acts as a co-ordinator and initiator of material processes. For example, in a task such as memory span, the CES coordinates the different mechanisms involved in the storage of the verbal items, including the ALS. Any individual task requires cognitive processes that draw on the resources of the CES. Placing two demanding tasks together is thought to exceed the capacity of the CES, resulting in mutual interference between tasks, with a subsequent decrement in performance. For example, Baddeley and Hitch (1974) combined remembering digits with sentence verification (that is, the phrase 'A follows B' was combined with the letters B-A, and the subject had to judge whether the phrase was true or false). When combined with only two digits, there was no interference in the speed or accuracy of the sentence verification task. However, when increased to six digits, there was substantial interference (Morris, 1994a).

Baddeley et al. (1991) suggest that the most extensively explored memory deficit is that associated with the amnesic syndrome, the gross impairment in long-term learning that occurs in Korsakoff patients, and in those patients with bilateral damage to the temporal lobes, hippocampus and diencephalon regions of the brain (Butters & Struss, 1989; Warrington & Weiskrantz, 1970). Such patients show grossly impaired learning of new material, whether visual or verbal, together with unimpaired short-term memory, as measured by digit span or by the recency effect in free recall (Baddeley & Warrington,

1970). The functioning of semantic memory may also be unimpaired, as indicated by retained knowledge of the meanings of words, and unimpaired speed of access of knowledge of the world, while the capacity to recollect events from well before the onset of the illness may also be relatively normal (Wilson & Baddeley, 1988).

The broad impairment in the capacity for new learning, coupled with a relative sparing of the recency effect in free recall, is shared by sufferers of Alzheimer's disease and the amnesic syndrome alike (Spinnler et al., 1988; Wilson et al., 1983). The memory deficit in Alzheimer's disease is more pervasive than that found in the amnesic syndrome and deficits in immediate memory span are shown by Alzheimer-type patients, whether tested verbally using the standard span procedure, or spatially using the Corsi Block Tapping technique (Spinnler et al., 1988). This deficit in Alzheimer-type patients in short-term or working memory has been explored in some detail by a number of researchers (Kopelman, 1985; Miller, 1973; Morris, 1984, 1986).

Morris (1994a) suggests that the most substantial deficits in Alzheimer-type patients are found on short-term memory tasks that require divided attention, including the variations on the task developed by Peterson and Peterson (1959). As Morris (1994a) explains, in this task the subject is presented with three verbal items (usually consonants or words) that have to be remembered after a delay during which he or she is distracted by a subsidiary task. Alzheimer-type patients show no impairment when the delay is left unfilled, but a severe impairment when distracted. The impairment has been found using a variety of distraction tasks, for example, reversing or adding pairs of digits or counting backwards in threes from 100 (Corkin, 1982; Kopelman, 1985; Morris, 1986; Sullivan, Corkin & Growden, 1986). In addition, the degree of impairment appears to be related to the severity of dementia (Corkin, 1982).

Studies of normal subjects and those with focal brain damage have split the ALS into a phonological short-term store (PSS) and an articulatory rehearsal mechanism (ARM) (Baddeley, 1992; Vallar & Baddeley, 1984). The rate at which Alzheimer-type patients can cycle verbal material through the ARM has been investigated (Hulme, Lee & Brown, 1993). A slower rate results in a reduction in the amount of material recycled, and hence a reduction in memory span (Morris, 1994a).

In normal subjects, the technique for measuring the rate of the ARM is for the subject to articulate overtly a series of verbal items, for example saying three words repeatedly (Baddeley, Thomson & Buchanan, 1975; Ellis & Hennelley, 1980). Morris (1984) and Hulme, Lee and Brown (1993) used this technique with mildly and moderately demented Alzheimer-type patients, respectively. Both groups of patients were significantly slower than matched elderly subjects. Despite this, there is a major problem of interpretation because of the difficulty that Alzheimer-type patients have in retrieving and holding the words in working memory, even if well-known sequences are used (Morris, 1994a). For example, in the Hulme, Lee and Brown (1993) study, the memory span long-word condition was on average only two words; yet in the equivalent articulation rate task, patients were required to articulate repeatedly two words, which they would frequently be unable to do (Morris, 1994a).

In Baddeley (1986) and Vallar and Baddeley (1984), another technique requires the subject to read a series of words as rapidly as possible, thus avoiding the difficulties in holding words in memory. Morris (1984) found no deficit in his Alzheimer-type patients with this reading measure. Therefore, if this task is regarded as the valid measure, the data suggest that the rate of recycling verbal material is undiminished in Alzheimer's disease.

Morris (1994a) suggests that it would be of interest to test patients who show more substantial loss of coherence, measured using PET or EEG, to discover whether or not they show a greater deficit on tests of executive function, such as the tasks used by Baddeley et al. (1991) and Baddeley et al. (1986), or the versions of the Peterson-Peterson tasks used by Morris (1986).

Clearly, there is scope for further research into memory models for Alzheimer's disease. Perhaps it is not surprising that research has concentrated on this most common form of dementia; however, it would be pleasing to see the results of these investments of time and money equally benefiting people with those less prevalent dementias that also have devastating effects on the sufferers, relatives and carers.

However, it seems that progress often follows this route, with minority sufferers having to wait for the benefits to filter down from the more prominent disorders. As well as public demand on research, the financial bodies that fund research into dementia very often have a vested interest, such as pharmaceutical companies, hence, it is not surprising that any benefits or 'spin-offs' have to be far-reaching to justify any financial outlay.

Biochemical and Anatomical Studies of Dementia

There have been numerous studies examining the causes and processes involved in the various types of dementia. A number of studies have focused on genetic factors possibly responsible for some of the clinical presentations of Alzheimer's disease (for example, Fischman et al., 1984) and the rarer types of dementias, such as Pick's disease. Research has also focused on biochemical pathways, changes to neuronal pathways (Whitehouse et al., 1981) and anatomical variations of brain structures (Miller, Alston & Corsellis, 1980). These studies are beyond the scope of this book, and the reader is referred to the specific (and often very technical) literature on each subject.

Psychological Stress in Caregivers

There is evidence that psychological stress adversely affects the immune system (Kiecolt-Glaser et al., 1995). In a study of 13 women caring for demented relatives, subjects underwent a 3.5 mm punch biopsy wound. Healing was assessed by photography of the wound and the response to hydrogen peroxide. 'Healing' in this method was defined as 'no foaming' of the hydrogen peroxide.

It was found that the carers' wound healing took significantly longer than in controls (48.7 versus 39.3 days, $p < 0.05$). The authors found that peripheral-blood leucocytes for caregivers produced significantly less interleuckin-1-beta mRNA in response to lipopolysaccharide stimulation than did controls' cells (Kiecolt-Glaser et al., 1995). Hence, stress-related defects in wound repair may have important clinical implications – for instance, for recovery from illness (Esterling et al., 1994) and surgery (Barbul, 1990). These findings are particularly relevant to 'relative' carers, where immunity changes have been previously found in spousal caregivers of dementing patients (Kiecolt-Glaser et al., 1991).

Early Onset Dementia Clinics

The National Service Framework for Older People (NHS, 2001) makes specific reference in Standard 7 to the need to action a review of current arrangements within the National Health Service (NHS) for the management of dementia in younger people. Furthermore, it suggests there is a need to implement local protocols across primary and secondary services. Previous studies have indicated the special issues for younger users of services, particularly those who have an early onset dementia (Luscombe *et al.*, 1998).

The Working Party of the West Sussex Health & Social Care NHS Trust sought to set up a clinic to assess, diagnose and initiate treatment for people under the age of 65 years who have dementia or cognitive dysfunction not attributable to head injury. This clinic was initially established for a 6-month trial period and operated under the title 'Adult Cognitive Assessment Team' (ACAT). This service was established and delivered by professionals from the 'Older Persons Mental Health Services' directorate who had particular interests and expertise in this area of care. Evaluation of patient outcome and of the impact of this new service provision informed service providers and planners. The success of the clinic has encouraged this NHS Trust to continue the clinic for a further period and to develop and improve upon service provision and patient care by additionally providing education and consultancy.

Initially, a survey of all general practitioners (GPs) in the Bognor Regis area (South Coast town in West Sussex between Portsmouth in the West and Chichester in the East) was undertaken to attempt to identify (a) the estimated or actual prevalence of dementia in the younger age group per practice, (b) the current treatment/referral options exercised by GPs in these circumstances, and (c) the specialist service requirements to address the needs of both this patient group and the primary care services. Results of this survey led to the establishment of an 'Early Onset Dementia Steering Group' that comprised members of the Trust, both clinicians and managers, as well as representatives from the private and voluntary sector. This group focussed on identifying actual and predicted local needs and, where possible, planning services around those needs.

Project Development

Lengthy consultation with users, carers, primary care services and secondary care professionals resulted in the formation of a core project group of professionals from Older Persons Mental Health services that have particular interest and expertise in the assessment, diagnosis and treatment of dementia. The recognition of unmet needs within the NHS Trust led to the development of a specialist outpatient clinic for younger people with cognitive dysfunction and/or suspected early onset dementia.

Demographic data showing a population of 175 000 (CPCS, 1997) reflected prevalence within the West Sussex region of approximately 230 patients under the age of 65 years with a known dementia. A brief survey of patients on active caseloads within the Chichester and Bognor Regis Community Mental Health Teams for Older People revealed a total of 23 known patients across the two areas. Whilst this is not a definitive indicator of need, it is probably a fairly accurate predictor of prevalence, taking into consideration that a significant number of people who have dementia in this younger age group will not be known to mental health services as a matter of course. Also, this figure does not take into consideration the number of patients who are actively known to the Working Age Mental Health Services or to neurology services, for example.

Elsewhere, similar services have been offered for some time, for example in London, the Alexandra Service, and also in Cambridge and in Greater Manchester (Baldwin, 2003). However, these services follow consultation with neurology and other professions and do not usually accept direct referrals from GPs or primary care staff. A review of services nation-wide for people under the age of 65 years with cognitive decline not attributable to head injury was limited. Whilst such services exist, some offering a range of interventions including day care and day hospital places, community support working or networks and continuing care facilities, there was no comparable service against which to objectively benchmark in terms of staffing, facilities, funding and resources and population demography. An eclectic model of service was therefore accepted, based on best practice in established services and resources within the Trust, and developed over the project period.

Memory clinics are established in many areas throughout the United Kingdom (Wright & Lindsay, 1995) as a clinically efficient and cost-effective process for assessing and rehabilitating out-patients who have specific memory impairment, and may complement organic day hospital provision as an effective alternative to present services, particularly for some out-patients with early-onset or mild to moderate dementia (Thompson, 1997; Thompson *et al.,* 2001) and head injury. Whilst this model of practice is not one that exists within the Trust, they are recommended as good clinical practice in the NHS National Service Framework for Older People (NHS, 2001) and a previous trial of running a memory clinic for people aged over 65 years in 2002 acted as a foundation in terms of experience upon which to base the Adult Cognitive Assessment Team (ACAT) service.

Development of this service was additionally guided by information and experience gained from a project which commenced in 1998, for one year, within Older Persons Mental Health Services in the previous Trust (Sussex Weald and Downs NHS Trust) which attempted to establish the effects of Donepezil on visual memory in those patients with mild to moderate Alzheimer's Disease (Thompson *et al.,* 2001). The project was funded by Pfizer Pharmaceuticals and involved the recruitment of a liaison (CATE - Cognitive Assessment, Treatment and Evaluation) nurse to support the prescription of Aricept to selected patients, the evaluation of assessment tools and the psychosocial impact of treatment with Aricept. The Consultant (in Old Age Psychiatry) and the Consultant Clinical Neuropsychologist for the CATE Project also led the ACAT service.

ACAT Services and Structure

The ACAT clinic was formed with the aim of responding directly to GP referrals, with the service tailored specifically towards assessment, diagnosis and treatment (where appropriate) of cognitive disorder by use of domiciliary and out-patient services, using inter-disciplinary expertise in the particular clinical, psychological and social needs of this care group. The clinic is distinct from other NHS regions in providing an inter-disciplinary review meeting prior to each clinic that considers both new referrals and the follow-up of patients seen in the preceding clinics. By developing maximum use of clinic time, patients referred to this service were seen at home within two weeks of referral and in the clinic within four weeks.

The team members included a consultant in old age psychiatry, specialist registrar in old age psychiatry, consultant neuropsychologist, senior occupational therapist, senior social worker, 3 community psychiatric nurses (G grades), clinical nurse specialist and management and clerical support. Furthermore, supplementary services such as physiotherapists and speech and language therapy services were involved in the core project development and were accessible as required once the clinic was operational, on a case-by-case basis.

The co-ordination of clinic appointments was undertaken by the manager who acted as the sole referral and entry portal into the project service. Once audit and demographic data had been collated, referrals were discussed at each inter-disciplinary meeting and processed from that point by the care co-ordinator identified, using the Single Assessment Process as the foundation data format.

A home visit by a clinician from the team enabled personal, social, medical and current history to be taken, in addition to introducing the service and explaining the process that would follow. Subsequent appointments to receive formal assessments from the consultant psychiatrist, consultant neuropsychologist and occupational therapist, spread over 3-4 clinic attendances, ensured that the most appropriate screening and assessment occurred. In addition to these reviews, home visiting continued throughout and the patient was subject to comprehensive physical screening.

Close links were developed with neurology services in the adjacent district general hospital, resulting in the seamless and rapid sharing of patient assessments both to and from this department. Access to MRI and CT scanning was more rapid in comparison to the usual out-patient referral processes, with all patients being seen within the time frame of the ACAT clinic duration itself.

Work is underway to develop an education and training component, maximising on the work already undertaken locally on informing GPs and primary health care teams of the role and purpose of the ACAT service, and a national publication addressing the educational and training needs of GPs (Coates, 1996). In addition, an education project is being proposed that will provide relatives of ACAT clinic attendees with advice on ways of identifying their own risk factors for cognitive decline or change, and practical ways in which their risks can be minimised. This will involve joint working with primary health care teams and Primary Care Trusts and is in keeping with current Department of Health initiatives in respect of improving the health of the population.

Further Reading

Deary, I.J., Hunter R., Langan, S.J. & Goodwin, G.M. (1991), 'Inspection time, psychometric intelligence and clinical estimates of cognitive ability in presenile Alzheimer's disease and Korsakoff's psychosis', *Brain*, 114, 2,543–54.

Fischman, H.K., Reisberg, B., Albu, P., Ferris, S.H., et al. (1984), 'Sister chromatid exchanges and cell cycle kinetics in Alzheimer's disease', *Biological Psychiatry*, 19, 3: 319–27.

Huppert, F.A. & Tym, E. (1986), 'Clinical and neuropsychological assessment of dementia', *British Medical Bulletin*, 42, 1: 11–18.

Kopelman, M.D. (1994), 'Working memory in the amnesic syndrome and degenerative dementia', *Neuropsychology*, 8, 4: 555–62.

Miller, E. (1971), 'On the nature of the memory disorder in presenile dementia', *Neuropsychologia*, 9, 75–81.

Morris, R.G. (1994a), 'Working memory in Alzheimer-type dementia', *Neuropsychology*, 8, 4: 544–54.

Philpot, M.P. & Levy, R. (1987), 'A memory clinic for the early diagnosis of dementia', *International Journal of Geriatric Psychiatry*, 2, 195–200.

Roth, M., Tym, E. & Mountjoy, C.Q. (1986), 'CAMDEX: a standardised instrument for the diagnosis of mental disorder in the elderly with special reference to the early detection of dementia', *British Journal of Psychiatry*, 149, 698–709.

Spinnler, H. & Della Sala, S. (1988), 'The role of clinical neuropsychology in the neurological diagnosis of Alzheimer's disease', *Journal of Neurology*, 235, 258–71.

Thompson, S.B.N. & Morgan, M. (1996), *Occupational Therapy for Stroke Rehabilitation* (2nd reprint), London: Chapman & Hall.

Chapter 12

Case Studies on Dementia and Learning Disability

People with Learning Disabilities and Dementia

People with learning disabilities are not exempt from illness. A common misconception is that having a learning disability is like having a *disease*, rather than a range of *abilities* that may be different or fewer than the wider population. The important point is that, like the general population, people with learning disabilities vary on an individual basis. Also, exposure to age-related conditions, such as senile dementia, becomes more probable as people live longer. People with learning disabilities can equally present with the signs of dementia.

Several attempts have been made in the past to describe this population (for example, Moss, Hogg & Horne, 1992) and a surprising number of articles were published in the early 1990s which addressed the issue of ageing as the primary subject of interest (Weisblatt, 1992).

However, the research literature has overwhelmingly focused on the proposed link between Down's syndrome and Alzheimer's disease (Olivcr & Holland, 1986; Delabar et al., 1987). Yet there is a need to examine the issues surrounding ageing in a broader context in order to plan and provide for specialist services for all types of learning disability (see Hogg, Moss & Cooke, 1988b).

In particular, there has been much controversy over the use of the Wechsler Adult Intelligence Scale and WAIS-R to assess people who have learning disabilities (Atkinson, 1991a). However, many researchers continue to compare populations according to IQ. Therefore, some sort of assessment of IQ seems inevitable in any study, if only to provide an approximate description of the abilities of clients being examined to enable comparisons.

Identifying Dementia in People with Down's Syndrome

In an attempt to address some of the complex issues surrounding the identification of dementia in people with learning disabilities, an examination was conducted by Thompson (1993a, 1993b) that considered a range of specific, standardised assessments. Following on from this, a neuropsychological test battery was compiled and tested (Thompson, 1994a), which comprised four well-known psychological assessment tools, and two new scales that had been previously tested only in a limited way. In addition, clients' biographical details and medical histories were collected (see Figure 12.1).

The remainder of the test battery comprised well-known psychological tests: the RCPM (Raven, Raven & Court, 1990), the WAIS-R (Wechsler, 1981a) and the MEAMS (Golding, 1989), which again was not originally designed for people with learning disabilities, but was used in this study.

The Study

Five male and three female clients diagnosed as having Down's syndrome were selected from people living in their own home or in voluntary organisation group homes. The average age of the clients was 51.1 years (range 44–63 years). Their average IQ was 51.2 (range 47–63), and all were asked if they wished to take part in the study, with the necessary consent (see Figure 8.5) and approval having been obtained from the local Ethics for Research Committee.

An explanation of how to complete each rating scale was given to the carer of each consenting client. Carers were asked to complete the HSSA and DMR for their clients, based on their knowledge of each client's abilities during the previous two months. The HAD was completed by the clinical psychologist, with the assistance of the carer, in an interview situation with the client (as explained above). The remaining tests were administered by the clinical psychologist on two separate occasions, usually beginning with the WAIS-R and followed by the MEAMS and RCPM on the second occasion (not more than seven days later). In addition, biographical details about each client were collected at this stage of the study, from carers' notes, medical notes (of the visiting doctor) and from appropriate carers and/or relatives.

Six months later, each client was approached to ask for permission to retest them. The HSSA and WAIS-R were not repeated at this stage, and the parallel version B of the MEAMS was administered. The RCPM, DMR and HAD were all administered as before. At 12 months, the DMR and HAD were again repeated to see if any changes had occurred. The following information was obtained from the test battery:

1. HSSA – total score and band reflecting the client's dependence;
2. DMR – sum of cognitive scores and sum of social scores;
3. HAD – total score for anxiety and total score for depression;
4. RCPM – total number of correct responses and percentile;
5. WAIS-R – verbal IQ, performance IQ and full-scale IQ;
6. MEAMS – total score and number of sub-tests passed;
7. Biographical details of each client tested.

Five out of eight clients were found to be in band 2 (and one client in band 1) of the HSSA, indicating that support was needed for several aspects of care, supervision and independence training (on average 3 or 4 hours in 24). Two clients fell into band 5, indicating greater dependence on carers (on average over 7 or 8 hours in 24), according to the guidelines for the HSSA (Hampshire Social Services, 1989).

All eight clients scored within the range 1–9 on the RCPM, placing them below the 5th percentile,which is well below that normally expected for the general population. Six out of eight clients showed score changes of at least 4 points on their sum of social scores in the DMR. These score changes were between each assessment for three clients, and between the second and third assessment for the remaining three clients. Using the IQ banding criteria for sum of social scores on the DMR (Evenhuis, 1992), two clients showed score changes in excess of 6.3, the value proposed for non-demented clients with Down's syndrome. Results of clients' sum of cognitive scores on the DMR indicated decline in three clients whose score changes were equal to or above 7 points between both the second and initial assessment, and also between the second and third assessment.

According to the IQ banding criteria for the sum of cognitive scores, two clients showed score changes above those of non-demented clients with Down's syndrome (5.8). Two clients were in a higher IQ banding to the remainder of clients, and no tabulated values have been provided by Evenhuis (1992) for either the Sum of Social Scores (SOS) or the Sum of Cognitive Scores (SCS) score changes in this IQ grouping.

All clients passed an average of 1.4 sub-tests of the MEAMS at the first assessment, and an average of 2.1 sub-tests on the second assessment six months later. Averages for total scores achieved on the MEAMS also varied: 14.3 (first assessment) and 16.0 (six-month assessment).

Only two clients showed levels of caseness for anxiety during the study, and two clients showed caseness depression. Two of the eight clients received medication during the study; these drugs were reviewed by the visiting general practitioner, and where possible, kept constant throughout the study. One client received phenytoin and the other carbamazepine, both for epilepsy. Neither client had episodes immediately prior to any of the assessments. Medication was considered to be managing the condition successfully in each case.

All eight clients in the study achieved scores on the WAIS-R equivalent to an IQ below 70; the average IQ of these clients (51.2) classifies a person, according to Wechsler (1981a), as being 'mentally deficient'. This term may not necessarily be of particular use, and indeed stigmatises people; however, it is perhaps not too surprising that these clients' performances were consistent with those they achieved on the RCPM, placing them at below the 5th percentile. This is also consistent with the finding that all of the clients had fairly high demands on the amount of support time required from carers, as seen by the HSSA scores and bands.

What is surprising is the relative, slight increases in some of the clients' total scores achieved on the MEAMS, although the number of sub-tests passed (which can be compared with normative tables) remain within those ranges normally expected of dementing persons in the general population. This finding could not be explained by practice effects, since the parallel version of the MEAMS had been administered. However, it is clear that at least six of the eight clients tested showed signs of declining skills generally, and that scores achieved on the DMR indicated signs of deterioration in cognitive and social skills in most cases. There was also evidence of score changes in the remaining two clients, although according to comparative data available from Evenhuis (1992), these changes were not significant. It is always possible, however, that greater score changes may have occurred in these clients at a further six-month re-test, hence showing possible signs of dementia.

Depression is often found in association with dementia, and as with the clients in this study, two clients exhibited signs normally associated with depression. However, one of these clients showed no signs of decline in social skills (DMR), but with the second client, the question could be raised of whether the presence of depression had confounded findings that indicated decline in social skills, or whether a differential diagnosis is necessary to explain findings for this client. It is difficult to discern the sensitivity of the DMR when used with depressed clients generally; indeed, Evenhuis (1992) has urged caution when interpreting results obtained in such situations. This still leaves us with the problem of discriminating between those clients who are dementing *only* from those that are depressed *only*.

This problem has been long debated, and presents itself predominantly when faced with assessing clients with limited communication and comprehension skills, such as those with some types of learning disability. Perhaps the only real answer to this problem is long-term behavioural observation of clients.

The DMR is a useful tool to indicate general areas of clients' skills that have declined; however, there is a need for a definitive assessment of depression for these clients in order to discriminate between the effects of depression and those of dementia. Such limitations to the use of the DMR make additional measures necessary: for example, the MEAMS can provide information that allows a subjective 'adjustment' to be made to the results of the DMR: the DMR may show a particular client to have global deficits, but specific deficits may be pin-pointed by using a direct client measure, such as the MEAMS, because the DMR is a carer-rated tool and cannot measure the client's skills directly, such as performance on a specific task.

The RCPM is also a global measure, and seeks to tap the client's intellectual abilities, providing the scorer with a percentile according to performance. The RCPM did not have ceiling or floor effects with the clients in the study; this is often a problem when using the WAIS-R (see Jones, 1987; Atkinson, 1991a, 1991b), particularly with people with learning disabilities, so the RCPM is a more popular choice of assessment. However, it does not identify a range of abilities like the WAIS-R, or provide a profile of skills for a given client.

The test battery which was presented attempts to provide the clinician with a convenient and relatively simple procedure for establishing and monitoring decline in clients with learning disabilities. It is not intended as a definitive measure of Alzheimer's disease (or multi-infarct dementia), but does provide a standardised format of monitoring decline in a range of cognitive functions over time. Generally, such tools are of considerable importance, especially when demands to assess elderly, dementing clients with learning disabilities seem to be on the increase.

Figure 12.1   Client's Biographical Details

Name:	**DOB:**
Keyworker:	**Place of residence:**

1	Cause of learning disability (if known):

2	Any problems with hearing and/or vision?

3	Any physical disabilities? (including year of stroke(s) if applicable)?

4	Any medical conditions (e.g. diabetes; epilepsy)?

5	Current medication (specify)?

6	Any special dietary requirements?

7	History of anxiety/depression/other mental health problems?

8	Recent loss/bereavement?

9	Any apparent memory problems?

   (a)	Fails to recognize familiar faces?
   (b)	Difficulty in recalling recent events?
   (c)	Difficulty in recalling past events?
   (d)	Forgets to keep appointments?
   (e)	Any other memeory problems (please state)?
   (f)	How long have these problems been apparent?

10	Interaction with others:

   (a)	Receives regular visits from friends or relatives?
   (b)	Types of friends: staff/residents/other (specify)?
   (c)	Can be him/herself with new people?
   (d)	Apparently anxious/hostile towards authority figures?

11	Social/education history

   (a)	Places of residence with approx dates (e.g. parental home, NHS home, voluntary organisation home)?
   (b)	Number of years' schooling?
   (c)	Type of school(s)?
   (d)	Able to read? (describe ability)?
   (e)	Able to write? (describe ability)?

12	Any additional information?

Neuropsychological Test Battery

The test battery consisted of the following:

1. Hampshire Social Services Assessment (HSSA);
2. Dementia Questionnaire for Mentally Retarded Persons (DMR);
3. Hospital Anxiety and Depression Scale (HAD);
4. Raven Coloured Progressive Matrices (RCPM);
5. Wechsler Adult Intelligence Scale – Revised (WAIS-R);
6. Middlesex Elderly Assessment of Mental State (MEAMS).

The two new scales that were used in the test battery were the HSSA (Hampshire Social Services, 1989), and the DMR, devised and first piloted by Evenhuis, Kengen and Eurlings (1990). The former of these scales addressed a number of self-care issues, and was designed as a questionnaire to be completed by the carer. For example, under the 'Independence' section, a sub-heading 'Eating' has several scored categories such as:

Eats all foods without any physical help at all. Not a messy eater. Uses knife, fork and spoon competently for appropriate foods. **SCORE 0**

Whereas for greatest independence under this section:

Requires physical help in carrying food from plate to mouth. Fed on soft foods. Sometimes will not open mouth and/or retains food in mouth without swallowing and/or regurgitates, and/or spits out food, and/or dribbles out food. **SCORE 8**

Other examples of scoreable categories include behaviour, amount of required supervision, and withdrawal from social activity. Responses to questions were scored and totalled, giving an overall 'band' that reflected the level of dependence or relative independence of the client. Scores from using this questionnaire could be used for grouping and comparing clients participating in the study according to their abilities/disabilities and dependence/ independence. Below is a list of categories covered:

1   Eating
2   Drinking
3   Communal meals
4   Hand washing
5   Managing in toilet
6   Continence/incontinence
7   Bathing
8   Teeth cleaning
9   Combing/brushing hair
10   Undressing
11   Dressing
12   Personal hygiene
13   Appearance:
     a)   skills
     b)   self-image
14   Moving about community
15   Use of transport
16   Use of community resources
17   Independent use of domestic rooms
18   Communication
19   Communication: verbal skills
20   Communication: non-verbal skills
21   Engagement in activities provided by carers
22   Social relationships
23   Physical disability
24   Withdrawal; excessive social/physical contact
25   Aggressive towards people
26   Self-injurious behaviour
27   Difficult/disruptive/destructive behaviours

The banding criteria is shown below:

Score Banding

Score	Band	Average staff support needed
0–30	1	Very minimal support needed (i.e. up to 1 hour in 24, often less).
31–60	2	Support to develop further independence, or support in specific areas, up to 2 hours in 24 on average.
61–110	3	Support for several aspects of care, supervision and independence training, on average 3 or 4 hours in 24.

111–150	4	Support for several aspects of care, supervision and in independence training, on average over 3-4 hours and up to 6-7 hours in 24; sleeping-in staff or waking staff needed.
151–200	5	Support needed in all major areas (on average over 7–8 hours in 24); sleeping-in staff or waking staff needed.
200–	6	24-hour support, including waking staff.

Summary:

1 = Practically/fully independent
2 = Fairly independent
3 = Some independence
4 = Little independence
5 = Very little/no independence
6 = Practically/fully dependent

The second new scale, the DMR was designed to assess the client's cognitive and social skills over time, and produced sets of scores from totalling the responses to each question that had been completed by the relative or carer of the client that reflected the client's relative independence or dependence upon others.

A significant decline in the difference scores from baseline to re-testing reflected a decline in cognitive and/or social functioning. From piloting the questionnaire in the Netherlands, Evenhuis (1992) produced sets of criteria for identifying scores that may indicate dementia in some of the clients in her study.

A third well-known scale, the HAD (Zigmond & Snaith, 1983), was used in a modified way to the original intentions of its authors (Figure 12.2). Since there is little in the way of standardised tests suitable for assessing depression in people with learning disabilities, this questionnaire was used by the carer, in conjunction with the clinical psychologist, in an interview situation. Questions were re-phrased, where appropriate, in order to pitch questions at a level of understanding appropriate to the individual client. It is appreciated that the HAD was originally administered as a self-rating tool, but it had become apparent in an earlier pilot study that the majority of clients interviewed either could not read or did not have sufficient ability to comprehend the questions in their original form. Therefore, in the absence of more suitable tests, an attempt was made to assess each client's psychological status with respect to depression and/or anxiety. This method was largely very satisfactory, since it usually confirmed knowledge about the client gained from other sources, such as from observations and recordings in the relevant notes, or carers' knowledge at that time. It was considered important to persevere in addressing this issue, since difficulties often arise when there is a differential diagnosis of depression and dementia (see Warren, Holroyd & Folstein, 1989; Yapa & Roy, 1990). Hence, provision for the HAD in the test battery was considered essential.

Figure 12.2   Anxiety and Depression Scale based on HADS

Q1 Do you feel tense or wound up?

---

3 Most of the time

2 A lot of the time

1 From time to time

0 Not at all

Q2 Do you still enjoy the things you used to enjoy?,

---

0 Definitely as much

1 Not quite so much

2 Only a little

3 Hardly at all

Q3 Do you get a sort of frightened feeling, as if something awful is about to happen?

---

3 Very definitely and quite badly

2 Yes, but not too badly

1 A little, but it doesn't worry you

0 Not at all

Q4 Can you laugh and see the funny side of things?

---

0 As much as you always could

1 Not quite so much now

2 Definitely not so much now

3 Not at all

Q5 Do worrying thoughts go through your mind?

---

3 A great deal of the time

2 A lot of the time

1 From time to time but not too often

0 Only occasionally

Q6 Do you feel cheerful?

3 Not at all
2 Not often
1 Sometimes
0 Most of the time

Q7 Can you sit at ease and feel relaxed?

0 Definitely
1 Usually
2 Not often
3 Not at all

Q8 Do you feel as if you are slowed down?

3 Nearly all the time
2 Very often
1 Sometimes
0 Not at all

Q9 Do you get a sort of frightenened feeling, like 'butterflies
   in the stomach?

0 Not at all
1 Occasionally
2 Quite often
3 Very often

Q10 Have you lost interest in your appearance?

3 Definitely
2 You don't take so much care as you should
1 You may not take quite as much care
0 You take just as much care as ever

Q11 Do you feel restless, as if you have to be on the move?

3 Very much indeed
2 Quite a lot
1 Not very much
0 Not at all

Q12 Do you look forward with enjoyment to things?

---

0 As much as you ever did
1 Rather less than you used to
2 Definitely less than you used to
3 Hardly at all

Q13 Do you get sudden feelings of panic?

---

3 Very often indeed
2 Quite often
1 Not very often
0 Not at all

Q14 Do you enjoy a good book or radio or TV programme?

---

0 Often
1 Sometimes
2 Not often
3 Not at all

KEY:
Anxiety questions - odd numbers; Depression questions - even numbers.
Anxiety/Depression Rating: 0–7 = normal range; 8–10 = borderline range; 11–21 = clinical range.

Cognitive Decline with Age in Down's Syndrome

It is recognised that all adults with Down's syndrome develop the neuropathological and neurochemical changes of Alzheimer's disease by their forties (Malamud, 1972; Roper & Williams, 1980; Wisniewski, Wisniewski & Wen, 1985). As Haxby (1989) states, only a minority of older Down's syndrome adults demonstrate clinically significant dementia (Haberland, 1969; Olson & Shaw, 1969; Reid & Aungle, 1974; Shapiro et al., 1986; Solitaire & Lamarche, 1966; Thase et al., 1983). It also seems to be the case that neuropsychological testing of older Down's syndrome adults indicates that behavioural changes may occur earlier, and may be more common than dementia (Dalton, Crapper & Schlotterer, 1974; Haxby, 1985; Schapiro et al., 1987). This suggests that the clinical diagnosis of dementia, based on caregiver reports and clinical neurological examination, may be insensitive to the early behavioural changes associated with Alzheimer's disease neuropathology in Down's syndrome.

Figure 12.3 Clients'/Relatives' Consent Form

Research into Dementia and People with Learning Disabilities

I am looking at how older people who live in the ********** area perform on various tasks.

    I hope that the results of these tests will tell me something about how ageing effects these results.

    I would be grateful if you would agree to take part in this research, which will mean answering some questions about yourself and doing some tasks.

    If you are not happy doing anything I ask you to do, at any time, you can stop immediately, and I will not ask you to do any further tests or answer any more questions.

    Do you understand what I am asking you to do? YES/NO

    Would you like to ask any questions, or explain anything to you? YES/NO

If you have understood what I am asking you to do and you
agree to take part, please sign this form here. Thank you.

Signed by

Witnessed by

(Position/Relationship to participant:)

However, not all researchers are convinced by this argument, and several have made attempts to identify dementia in Down's syndrome adults early on (for example, Evenhuis, 1992; Thompson, 1994a). It is acknowledged that dementia is difficult to diagnose in people with learning disabilities, because memory impairment and the beginning of disorientation is often not reported by patients themselves, nor often recognised by their caregivers (Lai & Williams, 1989; Evenhuis, Kengen & Eurlings, 1990; Wisniewski & Rabe, 1986).

As part of a comprehensive study, Das et al. (1993) looked at cognitive decline in people with Down's syndrome and considered specific tasks such as number finding, the Stroop Test (Trenerry et al., 1989), and a successive task, speech rate. In their sample, 46 people with Down's syndrome and 54 'mentally retarded people without Down's syndrome' were divided into four different age decades: 21–30 years, 31–40 years, 41–50 years and 51–60 years. A variety of tests were administered, including: the Dementia Rating Scale (DRS) (Mattis, 1988a), the Peabody Picture Vocabulary Test – Revised (PPVT-R) (Dunn & Dunn, 1981) and the Matrix Analogies Test (Naglieri, 1985).

The PPVT-R was selected for determining IQs because it is a verbal test, but without an explicit requirement for phonological coding or articulation, on which persons with Down's syndrome may still show variation on other cognitive tests which require the PASS processes (Planning, Attention, Simultaneous and Successive). Selection from the cognitive tests measuring the PASS cognitive processes were made from a recent version of a test battery (under development by the Riverside Publishing Co., Chicago) described in Naglieri and Das (1987). This paper also gives the rationale for constructing the tests from Luria's (1966) concepts of planning, attention, simultaneous and successive processes that have been presented and discussed in detail in a book by Das, Kirby and Jarman (1979) and several papers (Das, 1992; Naglieri & Das, 1988).

Das et al. (1993) found that the PASS measures, as found in the test battery, were preferable to the DRS because they were precise measures of processes and were theoretically supported. As measures of ageing in individuals with Down's syndrome as well as in non-Down's syndrome individuals, the tests were discriminative; decline in all of the tests were not shown for persons with Down's syndrome. If the older person with Down's syndrome had shown a decline in almost all cognitive tasks of the test battery, a possible cause could have been pervasive sensory impairment among persons with Down's syndrome.

As Das et al. (1993) point out, persons with Down's syndrome are known to have some hearing and visual problems, as well as problems in thyroid metabolism. However, examination of the various data does not provide any support for the possibility that persons with Down's syndrome are generally impaired at old age relative to the non-Down's syndrome group. Only three of the tasks (number finding, expressive attention and speech rate) demonstrate a disadvantage for persons with Down's syndrome over the age of 40. The first one is a visually-presented task, whereas the remaining two are presented auditorily; thus a pervasive sensory impairment would have resulted in poor performance in persons with Down's syndrome in the older group in the remaining seven tasks. Even considering 50 years of age as the dividing point, older persons with Down's syndrome did not show a relative disadvantage in six tasks.

Selective impairment in cognitive processing due to ageing does seem to be evidenced in Das et al.'s (1993) study by persons with Down's syndrome relative to non-Down's syndrome individuals. These cognitive processes require articulation, planning and attention, rather than coding of simultaneous and successive (visuospatial, auditory) information. For diagnosis of early signs of Alzheimer-type dementia, the tests that discriminate between individuals with Down's syndrome and non-Down's syndrome persons at 40 and then at 50 years of age seem to be particularly promising (Das et al., 1993).

Das et al. (1993) suggest that age-related decline among persons with Down's syndrome and non-Down's syndrome individuals ought to be studied longitudinally, as is done in the case of ageing in the non-learning-disabled population. The results of their study therefore need to be examined if and when longitudinal studies that involve at least three decades of life (the thirties, forties and fifties) become available. A cross-sequential design that combines longitudinal follow-up with cohorts for each decade as the longitudinal samples reach that decade would be the ideal study to determine the effects of ageing on cognitive processes (Das et al., 1993).

Central Executive System, Dementia and Learning Disability

Normal ageing brings with it certain changes to the higher mental or 'cognitive' functions (Allen, et al., 1997). Memory can also be affected (Craik, 1994), sometimes because the individual has failed to receive information correctly, or sometimes because it can no longer be effectively encoded or stored (Nyberg, et al., 1996). The effect of ageing on memory is very often one of the first of the cognitive functions to be noticed by others and can cause considerable distress to the individual and to relatives, close friends and carers. Deterioration in memory functioning is characteristic of dementia (Mitrushina, et al., 1995) but it can also indicate other dysfunctions which should always be considered in any assessment.

In a recent study, forty-one clients with learning disabilities (20 Down's syndrome, 21 non-Down's syndrome) were assessed using specially selected neuropsychological assessment tools at two time points separated by twelve months. Evidence for hypothesis 1 suggested that people with Down's syndrome show a greater decline in cognitive abilities with age, compared with other groups of people with learning disabilities.

A weak linear association ($p < .004$; $r = .625$; 2-tailed) between cognitive performance and social abilities was also found for the Down's syndrome clients, supporting hypothesis 2. Findings were explained in terms of the link between declining cognitive abilities and dementia and the documented evidence of language deficits in Down's syndrome.

Structural changes to the brain give rise to cognitive changes (Daigneault & Braun, 1993) that may be seen by others observing the individual. Anterograde memory functioning (often used to describe the every day memory functioning following an insult to the brain) has been attributed to the mammillary bodies deep within the brain structure. Following head injury, stroke or dementia, these tiny structures may become damaged (Kapur, et al., 1996) leading to loss of memory function. In normal ageing, the brain undergoes several structural changes including decreasing in size, flattening of the surface, and increasing amounts of intracranial space (Jernigan, et al., 1980). Other microscopic and biochemical changes occur as well as changes to the electrical activity (electrophysiological changes) within the brain (Zatz, et al., 1982). Verbal skills, particularly the well-learned skills of reading, writing, vocabulary, and word usage, tend to be maintained (Botwinick, 1977); and the general intellectual status of healthy older people, as measured by neuropsychological tests, tends to remain within normal limits through the eighth decade (Benton, et al., 1981).

Arithmetic ability is also generally stable among older people (Kramer & Jarvik, 1979). Arithmetic and memory tests that show decreased performance in older people, for example, Digits Backward of the Wechsler Adult Intelligence Scale-Revised (Wechsler, 1981), tend to reflect impaired concentration and mental tracking rather than decreased cognitive functioning (Parkin, *et al.*, 1995). However, a normal tendency for digit and letter span to be a little longer in the auditory than visual modality appears to increase with age (Kramer & Jarvik, 1979). Contrary to conventional belief, normal ageing processes do not affect the immediate memory span in older people (Nyberg, *et al.*, 1996).

Normal intellectual decline associated with old age shows up most strikingly in four areas of intellectual activity; these can be summarized as follows:

1. The primary, or working, memory capacity of intact older people differs little from that of younger adults (Erickson, 1978) except when the amount of material to be remembered exceeds the normal primary storage capacity of six or seven items, as in tests of supraspan (Craik, 1977). Older people use less effective learning procedures-less elaborative encoding (Fisk, *et al.*, 1997) and tend to show a greater differential between recall and recognition of learned material, particularly when the recognition tasks are easy (Botwinick & Storandt, 1974). Contrary to studies that indicate a progressive loss in recall of public events (Squire, 1974), Botwinick and Storandt (1980) reported that memory for remote events does not appear to change with the passage of time

2. Diminished ability for abstract and complex conceptualization typifies the intellectual functioning of older people (Botwinick,

1977). The more meaningful and concrete the presentation of reasoning problem, the greater is the likelihood that people will succeed at it (Botwinick, 1978).

3. Mental inflexibility, appearing as difficulty in adapting to new situations, solving novel problems, or changing mental set, characterizes intellectual performance failures of older age (Schaie, 1958). Some authors have suggested that apparent intellectual slowness in solving problems may be due to serial versus parallel processing. Evidence for slower serial processing was found in tests of older people as compared with younger participants (Ellis, *et al.*, 1996).

4. General behavioural slowing (Swearer & Kane, 1996) is a predominant characteristic of ageing that affects perceptual (Earles & Salthouse, 1995), cognitive (Thomas, *et al.*, 1977), and memory functions (Nyberg et al., 1996) as well as psychomotor activity (Benton, 1977; Welford, 1977). Accurate evaluation of an older person's poor performance on any timed test must depend on careful observation and analysis of the effect of time limits on the scores, for the score alone will tell little about the effects of slowing per se (Lezak, 1995).

There are of course several other conditions that might be confused with a diagnosis of dementia in older people. Some of these include paraphrenia, often defined as 'schizophrenia of late life', alcohol-related problems (such as Korsakoff's psychosis), and Parkinson's disease, the most common of which occurs in one or two people in every thousand (Goudie, 1993).

Memory failure is a common and significant problem in dementia, hence it is important to firs assess the extent to which it is a problem and for whom the problem is an obstacle.

It is widely accepted that different types of knowledge appear to be stored differently, so that, for example, knowing what a person ate for lunch (episodic memory) would be stored differently from knowing the word 'lunch' means a mid-day meal (semantic memory). Cohen and Squire (1981) have subsumed these terms under 'declarative memory' and reserve a further definition, termed 'procedural

Dementia and the Central Executive System

The definition of dementia generally accepted by clinical psychologists and psychiatrists is that outlined in DSM-IV (APA, 1994). In summary, it states that for a diagnosis of dementia, there should be demonstrable evidence of impairment in short-term and long-term memory. Impairment in short-term memory (ie inability to learn new information) may be indicated by an inability to remember three objects after five minutes. Long-term memory impairment (ie inability to remember information that was known in the past) may be indicated by an inability to remember past personal information (eg what happened yesterday; birthplace; occupation) or facts of common knowledge (eg past Prime Ministers; well known dates).

Dementia is commonly misunderstood to be a disease when in fact it may be the result of a number of factors, and in some instances it may be reversible. Stokes and Holden (1993) have described 'primary dementia' as an extensive, organic impairment of intellect memory and personality. It occurs in the absence of clouding of unconsciousness (ie without drowsiness) which is acquired, irreversible and progressive.

The single most common form of dementia is Alzheimer's disease which accounts for more than 50 per cent of cases of dementia in those over the age of 65 (Katzman, 1976). Typically, the onset is from 40 years of age onwards with insidious degeneration until death at about two to five years following onset (Jorm, 1990).

Each person with Alzheimer's disease will vary slightly in presentation according to personality. Emotional, behavioural and cognitive changes will also vary, but generally accepted by clinicians and researchers is a stage model which describes broad characteristics (Reisberg, 1983). In the first phase, the 'forgetfulness phase', there is usually difficulty in recalling recent events, and a tendency to forget where objects have been placed. Names of people and places, previously familiar, may be poorly recalled and a general disorientation persists and poor short-term memory. Abstract thinking, inability to concentrate on tasks and a marked lack of curiosity are also typical presentations. There may also be emotional changes such as anxiety and irritability and the 'new' or unexpected will be feared or disliked. Denial is also sometimes seen in presentation of people with Alzheimer's disease.

The second recognised phase is known as the 'confusional phase'. Increasingly poor attention span and a decline in generalised intellectual performance is seen with a deteriorating memory. Disorientation in place, word-finding difficulty and other changes to speech may be seen. Complex tasks are performed with difficulty, sometimes in a clumsy or inaccurate manner and often the skills the person learned last will be lost first. Hence the skills necessary for social independence and vocational skills are usually the first skills to be reduced or lost completely. Together with failing memory comes the concealment of these deficits by rationalising or confabulating events (ie providing an imaginary account of events or actions). Lack of interest in news and surroundings follows relatively quickly and can be extremely distressing to family and friends.

The third phase, the 'dementia phase', is characterized by a lack of purpose in the person's behaviour which appears disjointed and sometimes bizarre. Remaining intellectual and self-care abilities require constant supervision as people in this phase undergo further deterioration in memory capacity, calculating ability (dyscalculia) and aspects of language are severely affected and eventually lost. Constant assistance is required for self-care skills such as grooming, dressing, toileting and for feeding. A progressive physical wasting can also be seen which will mean help with walking. Sometimes one or two years of life will follow in an almost vegetative state until death.

In normal functioning, several types of information may be processed at once, possibly from a variety of sources. An example of this might be holding a conversation or driving a car. These types of activities break down relatively rapidly in patients with dementia, even at the early stages. Alberoni et al. (1992) reported that Alzheimer-type patients are particularly handicapped in keeping track of conversations involving several people. They also often have problems in remembering who said 'what' and 'when'.

This type of mental activity is successfully characterised by the Working Memory Model (Fig 12.6) developed by Baddeley and colleagues (Baddeley, 1986; 1992; Baddeley & Hitch, 1974). The model proposes a Central Executive System (CES) which functions to co-ordinate and schedule mental operations including the processing and immediate storage of information. This incorporates the notion of a 'scratch pad' system which holds and manipulates information simultaneously. The CES has limited resources, hence the decline in performance associated with trying to combine two attentionally demanding mental operations. A cluster of peripheral systems support the functioning of the CES. This includes a specialised Articulatory Loop System (ALS), responsible for recycling verbally encodable information, such as when a person tries to keep in mind a telephone number for a short period or understand a grammatically complicated sentence.

In the visuospatial domain, there is the visuospatial scratchpad (VSSP) which maintains visuospatial imagery. These components of the model are interacting continuously with the CES devoting varying degrees of processing resources to each component depending on the task. This is not the only model explaining sequencing and executive phenomena (Shallice, 1988; Furster, 1993), but it has provided a useful framework for studying cognitive impairment in dementia which has in part been characterised as a dysexecutive syndrome (Morris, 1986; Baddeley, *et al.*, 1986; Becker, 1988).

Figure 12.4   Schematic based on Baddeley's (1992) Working Memory Model

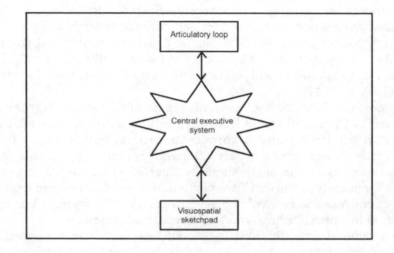

The peripheral systems of the Working Memory Model (Baddeley, 1992) are coordinated by the CES. The most extensively studied is the ALS which recycles verbal material in a relatively automatic fashion. For example, when remembering a string of digits, as in the digit span test of the Wechsler Adult Intelligence Scale Revised (Wechsler, 1981), the material is cycled continuously through the ALS to keep it in memory. A series of studies indicate that this system is unimpaired in Alzheimer's disease (Morris, 1984; 1987a,b; 1992). The evidence comes from experiments where patients are required to recall short lists of digits or words but the functioning of the ALS is suppressed by requiring them to mouth an irrelevant word (such as the word 'the'), effectively blocking articulatory rehearsal. 'Articulatory suppression' of this sort was found to have quantitatively the same effect on digits or words recall in Alzheimer's disease patients as in normal subjects. Thus, the equivalent loss of function without articulatory rehearsal shows the potency of the system to recycle verbal material is undiminished in Alzheimer's disease (Morris, 1984; 1987a,b; 1992).

The visual counterpart of the ALS is the visuospatial sketchpad which functions to retain visuospatial memory in immediate memory

(Baddeley, 1992). For example, if a person's attention is diverted momentarily from a visual scene, they will still maintain the memory of that scene for a short period. This ability helps the person maintain a sense of visual continuity when, for example, moving around the room. Although this ability has not been investigated extensively, there is evidence for significant impairment in visuospatial memory in Alzheimer's disease (Morris, 1994a). Firstly, patients with Alzheimer's disease have difficulty in a visual analogue of verbal span – the patient observes the experimenter tapping out a sequence on an array of nine blocks (or printed coloured squares as in the Wechsler Memory Scale Revised-Wechsler, 1988) in front of them and then has to immediately repeat the sequence of taps from memory. This block span performance has been found to be impaired consistently (Spinnler, *et al.*, 1988). Secondly, there is a measure known as the 'delayed matching to sample task' where an item is shown to the patient followed by a short delay followed by the same item with another or several others. The patient is required to pick out the item seen before. By varying the delay it is possible to see how fast memory for the item decays. Sahakian, *et al.* (1988) used a version in which a pattern was shown on a computer screen and the patient had to identify the pattern from four others. Early Alzheimer's disease patients were found to show more rapid forgetting than normal older controls. A later study by Money, *et al.* (1992) found a similar impairment using filled circles of different sizes, but Alzheimer's disease patients were impaired when there was no delay between presentation and choice and showed the same rate of forgetting as the controls. Both studies, therefore, showed a substantial impairment in the performance of Alzheimer's disease patients.

Baddeley et al. (1991) favours a localisationalist view; impairment in Alzheimer-type patients may be explained in terms of dysexecutive syndrome and frontal lobe dysfunction. This links the notion of the CES to the Norman and Shallice (1986) model of attentional control which assumes that most ongoing actions are controlled by establishing routines. The routines or 'schemas' are mutually inhibitory and can be triggered by environmental events. Where they are insufficient to generate appropriate activity, a higher-level system, the Supervisory Attentional System (SAS) comes into play which is involved in coping with novel circumstances or problem-solving activity (Morris, 1994b).

Shallice (1988) relates an impairment in the SAS to the difficulties patients with frontal lobe damage have in problem-solving. The conceptual link between the CES and the SAS has been introduced by Baddeley et al. (1991), who suggests that an SAS impairment also results in the reduced capacity to direct and control attentional resources. Thus an impairment in the SAS may be closely analogous to the dysexecutive syndrome seen in Alzheimer's disease. Indeed, Alzheimer's disease patients do have damage to their frontal lobes (Morris, 1994b).

The Study

A link has been known for some time between people who have the neuropathology of DS and their subsequent development of clinical signs, associated with Alzheimer's-type dementia. Less is known about the effects of dementia on non-DS persons with learning disabilities and whether there is any difference when compared with DS individuals. However, there is substantial evidence to show that cognitive abilities may decline with the onset and progress of dementia.

Hypothesis 1: Do people with DS show a greater decline in cognitive abilities with age compared with other groups of people with learning disabilities?

Hypothesis 2: Do cognitive abilities decline over time together with social abilities?

Materials

Wechsler Adult Intelligence Scale-Revised (WAIS-R) (Wechsler, 1981); Raven Coloured Progressive Matrices (RCPM) (Raven, *et al.*, 1995); Middlesex Elderly Assessment of Mental State (MEAMS) (Golding, 1989); Hampshire Social Services Assessment (HSSA) (HSS, 1989). (To make the HSSA more user-friendly and less confusing to use, zero scoring items which were indicated by an asterisk in the original version, were changed to a zero and normal typeface headings were changed to bold typeface).

Golding and others have discussed the use of the MEAMS dementia screening tool (Golding, 1989; van Belle, *et al.*, 1990). In the MEAMS manual, Golding states that it systematically surveys the major areas of cognitive performance, namely, orientation, name learning, comprehension, remembering pictures, arithmetic, spatial construction, fragmented letter perception, unusual views, usual views, verbal fluency, and motor perseveration. Score 10-12 are 'normal' and scores 8 or 9 are 'borderline range'. Although she states in her three-level criteria, score performance, she does not report test-retest data using the parallel version of the test. Hence, the actual amount of discrepancy seems to be very dependent on the population studied (Powell, *et al.*, 1993).

Dementia Questionnaire for Mentally Retarded Persons (DMR) (Evenhuis, 1992a); Hospital Anxiety and Depression Scale (HAD) (Zigmond & Snaith, 1983); information sheets for participants; sheets for the collection of clients' biographical details, and consent forms.

Sample

(i)   'Down's Syndrome' (DS)-Group 1

Eleven male and 9 female clients (DS1-DS20) with an average age of 47.25 years (sd = 1.33) and range of 35-63 years (Table 12.1) were randomly selected from the consultant psychiatrist's list of people from the South of the United Kingdom. All clients agreed to participate in the study. All clients were diagnosed by the consultant psychiatrist as having Down's Syndrome and were found to have an average full-scale IQ on the WAIS-R of 51.90 (sd = 1.21) and range of 47-63 IQ points. Scores of clients' performances on the RCPM placed the majority of clients in the "less than the 5th percentile" (Raven, *et al.*, 1995) band, indicating low intellectual ability.

Table 12.1   Group 1: Summary of HSSA and WAIS-R Results

CLIENTS (m=male; f=female)	HSSA Score	Band	AGE	WAIS-R (IQ) Verb.	Perf.	F-Scale
MEAN	37.83	1.65	47.25	54.75	59.00	51.90
SD	4.86	3.03	1.33	1.32	1.12	1.21

Key: *Verb. = Verbal IQ*
         Perf. = Performance IQ
         F-Scale = Fullscale IQ
         SD = Standard Deviation

HSSA scores of the majority of clients (13) fell into band 1, indicating "very minimal support needed (i.e, up to 1 hour in 24, often less)" (HSS, 1989; p.7). Five clients fell into band 2, and two clients fell into band 5; the latter indicating "support needed in all major areas (on average over 7/8 hours in 24). Sleeping-in staff or waking staff needed". Mean band: 1.65; sd: 3.03; range: 1-5.

(ii)　　　*'Non-Down's Syndrome' (NDS)-Group 2*

Ten male and 11 female clients (NDS1-NDS21) with an average age of 56.43 (sd = 1.21) years and range of 45-68 years (Table 12.2) were randomly selected from the consultant psychiatrist's lists of people from the South of the United Kingdom. All clients were diagnosed by the consultant psychiatrist as having a learning disability other than DS and fell into the following categories: prenatal abnormality/ illness (eg rubella; meningitis); perinatal trauma (eg anoxia; cerebral palsy); or metabolic (eg phenylketonuria). None of the clients had a genetically acquired learning disability.

All agreed to participate in the study. Clients were found to have an average full-scale IQ on the WAIS-R of 59.19 (sd = 1.17) and range of 51-69 IQ points. Scores of clients' performances on the RCPM placed the majority of clients in the "less than the 5th percentile" band, indicating low intellectual ability; five clients were placed in the higher 25th percentile ability band.

HSSA scores ot ten clients fell into band 3, indicating "support for several aspects of care, supervision and independence training, on average 3 or 4 hours in 24" (HSS, 1989; p. 7). Six clients fell into band 1, four clients fell into band 2, and one client fell into band 4; the latter indicating "support for several aspects of care". Mean band: 2.29; sd: 1.75; range: 1-4.

Controls

Each client was his/her own control. Individual's scores obtained at the first assessment were compared with their own scores at each subsequent assessment. In this way, it was possible to identify those clients who showed probable decline in cognitive abilities, as reflected in their change in scores over time.

Procedure

Permission and approval for this study was granted by the local ethics committees. Consent was obtained from those people in charge of the caring establishments approached as well as from individual clients. The following summarises information obtained from each assessment:

Table 12.2   Group 2: Summary of HSSA and WAIS-R Results

CLIENT (m=male; f=female)	HSSA Score	Band	AGE	WAIS-R (IQ) Verb.	Perf.	F-Scale
MEAN	55.19	2.29	56.43	61.90	63.43	59.19
SD	2.29	1.75	1.21	1.18	1.14	1.17

Key: Verb. = Verbal IQ
Perf. = Performance IQ
F-Scale = Full-scale IQ
SD = Standard Deviation

First Assessment

1. HSSA-total score and band reflecting the client's dependence;
2. DMR-sum of cognitive scores and sum of social scores;
3. HAD-total score for anxiety and total score for depression;
4. RCPM-total number of correct responses and percentile;
5. WAIS-R-verbal IQ, performance IQ and full-scale IQ;
6. MEAMS-total score and number of subtests passed;
7. Biographical details of each clients tested.

Second Assessment (at 12 months)

1. DMR-sum of cognitive scores and sum of social scores;
2. HAD-total score for anxiety and total score for depression;
3. RCPM-total number of correct responses and percentile;
4. MEAMS (version B)-total score and number of subtests passed.

Results

Scores obtained using the RCPM, reflected performances below the 5th percentile in all but one case for each client group (DS17 & NDS9), which were both at the 10th percentile. Test scores obtained for each group of clients were compared. No statistically significant differences were found between the measures: Age, WAIS-R, Full-scale IQ and HSSA thus confirming the similarity of ability profiles of the two groups.

Test scores obtained at assessments 1 and 2 were compared. For the DS clients (Table 12.3), all except the MEAMS Total scores were found to be significant. After controlling for the effects of 'anxiety' and 'depression' by partialling out these HAD scores, the following were found to be significant (Table 12.4): the 'sum of social scores' of the DMR (p < .001, HAD Anxiety out; p < .003, HAD Depression out). No significant interaction effects were found.

Table 12.3   Group 1: Comparison of Test Measures between Assessments 1 and 2

Variable	Mean	SD	SE	df	F	p
DMR (SOS)	16.70	9.88	2.21	19	132.229	<.001
DMR (SCS)	3.54	1.66	0.37	19	7.535	<.04
MEAMS Tot.	25.40	15.00	3.35	19	1.823	.202 (ns)
MEAMS Sub.	1.61	0.86	0.19	19	23.202	<.001
HAD Anxiety	1.39	0.24	5.42E-02	19	4.901	<.01
HAD Dep.	1.34	0.86	0.19	19	18.127	<.001

Table 12.4   Group 1: Comparison of Test Measures between Assessments 1 and 2 Controlling for 'Anxiety' and 'Depression'

Variable	Anxiety Out			Depression Out		
	df	F	p	df	F	p
DMR (SOS)	14	160.541	<.001	14	84.416	<.003
DMR (SCS)	15	4.668	.190 (ns)	15	10.648	.089(ns)
MEAMS Tot.	16	1.192	.519 (ns)	16	1.458	.580 (ns)
MEAMS Sub.	2	58.579	<.001	2	33.184	<.001

Key to Tables 3 & 4:

SD = Standard deviation
SE = Standard error
DMR = Dementia Questionnaire for Mentally Retardred Persons
SOS = Sum of social scores of DMR
SCS = Sum of cognitive scores of DMR
MEAMS Tot. (Sub.) = Middlesex Elderly Assessment of Mental State total scores (subtests passed)
HAD Dep. = Hospital Anxiety and Depression Scale depression score
ns = Not significant

Table 12.5 **Group 2: Comparison of Test Measures between Assessments 1 and 2**

Variable	Mean	SD	SE	df	F	p
DMR (SOS)	14.05	9.34	2.04	20	1.255	.396 (ns)
DMR (SCS)	2.46	1.84	0.40	20	3.388	<.02
MEAMS Tot.	26.62	13.37	2.92	20	4.109	<.05
MEAMS Sub.	1.67	0.61	0.13	20	19.693	<.001
HAD Anxiety	1.32	0.38	8.32E-02	20	0.928	.546 (ns)
HAD Dep.	1.17	0.98	0.21	20	2.978	<.05

Key:
SD = Standard Deviation
SE = Standard Error
DMR = Dementia Questionnaire for Mentally Retardred Persons
SOS (SCS) = Sum of social (cognitive) scores of DMR
MEAMS Tot. (Sub.) = Middlesex Elderly Assessment of Mental State total scores (no. subtests passed)
HAD Dep. = Hospital Anxiety and Depression Scale depression score
ns = Not significant

For the non-DS clients (Table 12.5), all except the 'sum of social scores' of the DMR and Anxiety scores were found to be significant. After partialling out the HAD scores (Table 12.6), the following were found to be significant: the 'sum of cognitive scores' of the DMR ($p < .05$, HAD Anxiety out); and the MEAMS number of sub-tests passed ($p < .001$), HAD Anxiety out; $p < .001$, HAD Depression out). No significant interaction effects were found.

The decline in cognitive scores on the DMR for the DS group was greater than that of the non-Down's syndrome group ($p < .04$; df = 1; F = 7.630). These findings support hypothesis 1 which suggests people with DS show a greater decline in cognitive abilities with age.

Examining Linear Relationships within the Data

For the DS clients, an association was found between the 'sum of social "difference" scores' of the DMR with the MEAMS number of subtests passed "difference" scores ($r = .625$; $p < .004$; 1-tailed). After controlling for HAD Anxiety and HAD Depression scores, this association remained significant ($r = .522$; $p < .04$; 1-tailed) (Table 12.7). No statistically significant relationship was found with the 'sum of cognitive "difference" scores. For the non-DS clients, these measures were not found to be significantly associated.

Table 12.6   Group 2: Comparison of Test Measures between Assessments 1 and 2 Controlling for 'Anxiety' and 'Depression'

Variable	Anxiety Out			Depression Out		
	df	F	p	df	F	p
DMR (SOS)	13	2.467	.163 (ns)	13	1.106	.493 (ns)
DMR (SCS)	12	6.008	<.05	12	3.203	.082 (ns)
MEAMS Tot.	14	3.080	.143 (ns)	14	2.743	.170 (ns)
MEAMS Sub.	2	14.366	<.001	2	14.081	<.001

Table 12.7   Partial Correlation Coefficients for Group 1 before and after Controlling for 'Anxiety' and 'Depression'

Variable	Significance Level					
	Before			After		
	df	r	p	df	r	p
DMR (SOS) difference scores with MEAMS Sub. difference scores	18	0.625	<.004 (<.003)	14	0.522	<.04 (<.02)
DMR (SCS) difference scores with MEAMS Sub. difference scores	6	0.580	.132 (ns)	2	0.934	.066 (ns)

Key to Tables 12.6 & 12.7:
DMR = Dementia Questionnaire for Mentally Retarded Persons
SOS = Sum of social scores of DMR
SCS = Sum of cognitive scores of DMR
MEAMS Tot. (Sub.) = Middlesex Elderly Assessment of Mental State total scores (no. subtests passed)
r = Partial correlation coefficient
ns = Not significant
(Note: Parentheses indicate 1-tailed testing; otherwise 2-tailed testing shown.)

These findings suggest that for the DS clients, there is a weak association between the social ability scores of the DMR with the scores of the MEAMS. This supports hypothesis 2 suggesting that both cognitive abilities (as measured by the MEAMS, for example) and social abilities (as measured by the DMR, for example) decline over time.

Discussion

Social Abilities

On comparing data obtained from both client groups, a statistically significant difference was found in the 'sum of social "difference" scores' of the DMR between assessments 1 and 2 (p < .002). Although the majority of HAD scores for clients fell within the 'normal' range (i.e., below 8 points), the effect of controlling for these scores was evidenced when they were partialled out in data analyses: p < .02 (after HAD Anxiety was partialled out), and p < .003 (after HAD Depression was partialled out). Therefore, the level of statistical significance of this finding was reduced following controlling for the HAD scores.

It it perhaps not surprising to find that anxiety and depression are related to the level of social abilities. This finding tends to support what is already known about the influence of depression and anxiety levels on clients' abilities (Yapa & Roy, 1990; Agbayewa, et al., 1991) and it is suspected that although the HAD scores for the majority of clients in the study were not in the 'borderline' or 'caseness' range, some level of anxiety and/or depression does seem to affect a person's capabilities and performance in the area of social skills.

In addition, the DS clients showed a greater score difference between assessments 1 and 2 in the 'sum of social scores' than the non-DS clients. It is known that people with DS very often have expressive (Young & Kramer, 1991) and receptive (Hartley, 1982) language difficulties. It is proposed that the differences in scores between people with DS and other learning difficulties may be due partly to the known differences in understanding language in the ability for expressive language. Since language is important in the development of social abilities, this impediment may well account for the difference in social abilities seen between the two client groups.

Cognitive Abilities

On comparing scores obtained on the MEAMS number of subtests passed, 4 of the 20 DS clients showed decline, 7 clients slightly improved, and 9 showed no change in their scores. Of the 21 non-DS clients, 9 showed a decline in scores, 1 slightly improved, and 11 showed no change. A significant score change was found (p < .001) in the DS clients suggesting that cognitive abilities co-vary over time.

It may well be that decline in social abilities occurs before decline in cognitive abilities in this population, or possibly that the latter is more subtle and difficult to measure in these clients. A decline in social skills, for example, may be more noticeable and easily assessed because of the person's withdrawal from socialising or because of decreased interaction with care staff. Little is known in the learning disability population about the rate of decline or whether decline in cognitive abilities occurs in the same way as it seems to occur in people without learning disabilities who are dementing; although, rate of cognitive decline with age in people who are not dementing, who have DS or "other" learning disabilities seems to be indistinguishable from one another (Das, *et al.*, 1993).

For the DS group, only two clients (DS11 and DS12) scored above 7 (number of subtest passed) at assessment 1. At retest (assessment 2), no clients scored above 7; hence, according to Golding (1989) this would place all these clients in the third (lowest) category where 'more detailed investigation' is recommended. It is curious to note the slight improvement in some scores though all scores were still below the 7-point cut-off stated by Golding (1989) with a mean score for the "differences" between assessments 1 and 2 (for all DS group data) of only 0.30, and a very large variance (standard deviation = 13.33).

For the non-DS group, the mean of scores for the MEAMS number of subtests passed with higher than for the DS group with a mean for these "difference" scores of − 0.57 and a lower variance and less spread than for the DS group (standard deviation = 3.51). Although no statistical difference was found between the two client groups on the MEAMS number of subtests passed, it would seem that of the two client groups, more clients in the non-DS group showed a deterioration in their performance on the MEAMS than did the DS group. It is possible that cognitive abilities were more developed in the non-DS clients and may have been more prone to the debilitating effects of dementia.

Cognitive impairment is salient in dementia in the non-learning disabled population. In particular, executive phenomena have received recent interest which have led to the development of a new assessment measure, the Behavioural Assessment of the Dysexecutive Syndrome (Wilson, *et al.*, 1996). Shallice (1988) and Furster (1993) have also explained the cognitive impairment in dementia in terms of a failure in sequencing and executive phenomena, such as the ability to organise and plan, an Morris (1984; 1986), and others, have described this is in terms of a 'dysexecutive syndrome'. Yet, there is still a lack of substantive evidence of such familiar impairments in people with learning disabilities who have dementia, although it is thought that people with DS tend to decline cognitively (Das, *et al.*, 1993), but the rate of decline seems to vary considerably. Neither has this been particularly well documented, nor have there been well-matched comparisons with non-DS learning disabled people with a diagnosis of dementia.

The cognitive impairment seen in people with dementia may also be considered in terms of Baddeley's (1986) Central Executive System(CES). A breakdown in one of the supporting systems to the CES, the Articulatory Loop System (ALS), responsible for recycling verbally encoded information, may account for the difficulties that learning disabled people (particularly DS) tend to have with tasks that require intact verbal memory functioning. Language difficulties also impact on tests of cognitive functioning that require verbal responses, for example, the 'verbal' subtests of the WAIS-R and the world fluency subtest of the MEAMS. However, despite some reports of articulatory rehearsal impairments in Alzheimer's disease (eg Hulme, *et al.*, 1993), impressive evidence comes from 'articulatory suppression' tasks (Morris, 1992) which tend to suggest that perhaps the ALS is not implicated in dementia since, particularly Alzheimer-type patients, perform equally well to normal controls. This finding may lend support to the lack of a significant difference in this study between the two client groups in their MEAMS scores.

In the visuospatial domain, the visuospatial sketchpad (Baddeley & Hitch, 1974; Baddeley, 1986), which maintains visuospatial imagery, is thought to be operative in tasks requiring spatial construction (Sahakian, *et al.*, 1988); to some extent, this applies to the visuospatial subtest of the MEAMS. Visuospatial ability is thought to be significantly impaired in people with dementia; however, it has not been investigated extensively (Morris, 1994a).

Examining Linear Associations between Measures

It does seem to be the case that cognitive abilities (as measured by the DMR 'sum of cognitive "difference" scores') are not associated in a linear manner with scores on the MEAMS. No significant linear relationship was found for date of either client group. However, a significant (though weak) linear relationship was found between the DMR 'sum of social "difference" scores' with the MEAMS number of subtests passed "difference" scores (r = .522; p < .04; 1-tailed; after controlling for HAD scores) for the DS group. Hence, it is suggested that if social abilities decline in people with learning disabilities (particularly those with DS) then this decline may correlated with their performance on the MEAMS.

Examination of data for each client group individually, revealed that for the DS group, there was a significant difference between assessments 1 and 2 on the DMR 'sum of social scores' (p < .001). A significant difference remained following the partialling out of HAD scores. These scores were not significant for the non-DS group. Hence, this is strong evidence for suggesting that social abilities significantly co-vary over time in people with DS, thus "partially"supporting hypothesis 2, since evidence was only found for the Down's Syndrome group.

Data from the non-DS clients also supported the view that cognitive abilities (as measured by the DMR 'sum of cognitive scores') decline over time (p < .05; HAD Anxiety partialled out). Although, when HAD Depression was partialled out, these scores were not significant. It is possible that some of these clients suffered from mild depression (whether or not as a consequence of dementia) and hence their performance on tests of cognitive abilities were affected.

These data tend to partially support hypothesis 2 in that cognitive abilities seem to co-vary over time for both groups of clients.

Problems of a Differential Diagnosis

In terms of the HAD scores between assessments 1 and 2, it was found that both HAD Anxiety and HAD Depression scores co-varied over time, though more significantly in the DS group. This finding can possibly be explained in terms of people's frustrations and low mood which has been evidenced in the non-learning disability population who are dementing (Lamberty & Bieliauskas, 1993). However, it is not known whether the presence of depression is more salient in people with DS versus other learning disabilities with or without dementia. However, it is important here to address the problem of a differential diagnosis, particularly between dementia and depression. HAD scores were found to be in the borderline range with the majority falling into the 'normal' category. It is recognized that discriminating between dementia and depression in the non-learning disability population is difficult but not impossible, for example, using the Beck Depression Inventory (Beck & Steer, 1987) in conjunction with measures of social and cognitive abilities and the clinical interview.

However, in the learning disability population, it is increasingly difficult when language and comprehension is limited. Despite these difficulties, it is believed that the modified use of the HAD (in an interview situation) and the fact that third parties (namely carers) also contributed to the data pool (by completing the DMR, for example), helped to strengthen the methodology implemented, and hence produce valid results. In addition, biographical data helped to confirm that none of the clients had been observed to be depressed prior to the study nor did any of them have a known history of depression or low mood swings.

Recently, the link between probable Alzheimer's disease and stroke has been reported (Nash, 1997). Studying nuns from a convent in the United States, Snowdon believes that nuns who suffered a stroke also increased their chance of developing Alzheimer's disease. This supports the view that Alzheimer's disease should perhaps be studied together with vascular disease, particularly transient ischaemic attacks, multi-infarcts and cerebrovascular disease.

Conclusions

A statistically significant difference (p < .001) was found in the MEAMS number of subtests passed (i.e., "cognitive abilities") between assessments for the DS and non-DS clients. This decline was greater in the DS clients. This supports hypothesis 1, which proposed that the DS clients showed a greater decline in cognitive abilities with age, compared with other groups of people with learning difficulties.

Several explanations were proposed for the differences found between the two client groups; namely, the well-documented difficulties with language (comprehension and expression) in people with DS may affect their social abilities. Also, in comparison with Evenhuis' (1992a,b) samples, decline in social abilities has been found to be associated with a dementing process particularly in people with DS.

Evidence was found to support hypothesis 2 which suggested that cognitive and social changes co-vary over time in these two older populations. Social and cognitive abilities tended to co-vary in the non-DS clients whilst cognitive abilities tended to co-vary in the non-DS clients. These findings were discussed in terms of the 'dysexecutive syndrome' (Shallice, 1988; Furtster, 1993; Wilson, *et al.*, 1996) which suggests that cognitive impairment in dementia occurs because of a failure in sequencing and executive phenomena, such as planning and organising. Impairments possibly due to changes in visuospatial ability were also discussed in terms of Baddeley's (1986) 'visuospatial sketchpad' which maintains visuospatial imagery as part of the Central Executive System.

Data were also examined for linear associations. Although a significant association was found between the MEAMS number of subtests passed "difference" scores and the DMR 'sum of social "difference" scores' (p < .05), this correlation was weak (r = .5219). It was suggested that declining social abilities of DS clients may be weakly associated with performance on the MEAMS.

Finally, it was suggested that further longitudinal studies should be conducted that compared different forms of dementia, and particularly with vascular disorders such as multi-infarcts and stroke.

Conclusions about Studies on Learning Disabilities and Dementia

Studies into the effects of ageing on people with learning disabilities are ever-increasing. Much can be learned from studying people with Down's syndrome. However, this type of research is only useful if the information obtained can be fed back to participants and carers in order to improve their long-term care.

As the population of older people grows, the demand for caring for older people with learning disabilities also grows. Therefore, it is time to invest in research for these people, as they will form a substantial proportion of our growing older population in time to come.

Further Reading

Collacott, R.A. & Cooper, S. (1992), 'Adaptive behaviour after a depressive illness in Down's syndrome', *Journal of Nervous & Mental Disease*, 180: 468–70.

Evenhuis, H.M. (1992), 'Evaluation of a screening instrument for dementia in ageing mentally retarded persons', *Journal of Intellectual Disability Research*, 36: 337–47.

Haxby, J.V. (1989), 'Neuropsychological evaluation of adults with Down's syndrome: Patterns of selective impairment in non-demented old adults', *Journal of Mental Deficiency Research*, 33: 193–210.

Kiecolt-Glaser, J.K., Marucha, P.K., Malarkey, W.B., Marcado, A.M., et al. (1995), 'Slowing of wound healing by psychological stress', *Lancet*, 346: 1,194–6.

Light, E., Niederhe, G. & Lebowitz, B.D. (eds) (1994), *Stress Effects on Family Caregivers of Alzheimer's Patients*, New York: Springer.

Thompson, S.B.N. (1993b), *Eating Disorders: A Guide for Health Professionals*, London: Chapman & Hall, 194–240.

Chapter 13

Future Directions for People with Dementia

Screening Older People for Dementia

In the 1980s, various researchers proposed screening older people for the early detection of disorders such as dementia. At this time, it was probably seen as a possible solution to the problem being faced – a steadily increasing population of older people, and hence an increasing number of people with dementia. The scope for the early detection of dementing disorders in older people has been reviewed (for example, Cooper & Bickel, 1984). The authors concluded that while there was an urgent need for psychogeriatric screening methods, such methods were still at an early experimental stage. Indeed, no major progress in this field can be expected unless early case detection can somehow be integrated with methods of systematic surveillance of the at-risk older population. The practical problems, as well as the ethical dilemmas, still prevail.

In the 1990s, researchers re-examined the use of well-known screening tools such as the Mini-Mental State Examination (Folstein, Folstein & McHugh, 1975); Braekus (1995) discovered that individuals scoring 24–25 (around the cut-off point) are at high risk of developing dementia within three years.

Collecting Research Data

A number of studies have considered ways to monitor people for dementia. However, a growing problem is also the many associated problems that may manifest in the older population. In order to monitor Older Peoples Mental Health Services (OPMHS), a survey was conducted within the West Sussex Health & Social Care NHS Trust by the Clinical Neuropsychology Services to compare service uptake against guidelines set out in the National Service Framework for Older People and the Department of Health's 'Treatment Choice in Psychological Therapies and Counselling'.

   A questionnaire was completed for all new referrals to OPMHS in Chichester, Midhurst, Bognor Regis, Crawley and Horsham, by the clinical team to record whether or not psychological therapies had been appropriately considered for patients. Additional information was included: where psychological services were appropriate, how they were progressed. These data were collected between April and September 2002.

Results

In total, 68 questionnaires were completed for 118+ new referrals (see: Note 1) to OPMHS.

Q1. Does the patient require psychological help?	No. of responses	% of responses
Yes	28	42
No	40	58

Note 1: Data only for the total number of in-patients referred during this period (118) was available at this time. Hence, the total number will be greater.

Figure 13.1   Percentage of People requiring Psychological Help

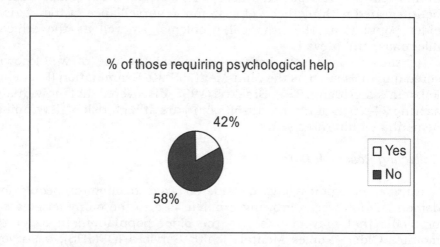

Q2. If NO, please specify reason:	Responses	%
Not clinically indicated / appropriate	11	28
Blank	7	18
Depression being treated / recovering / mild	4	10

Dementia / end stage dementia	5	12
Mild cognitive deficits	2	5
Emergency referral / acute depressive crisis	2	5
Requires social care / respite / assessment for equipment	7	18
Has private counsellor	1	2
Having ACI Therapy only	1	2

Figure 13.2   Percentage of People not requiring Psychological Help

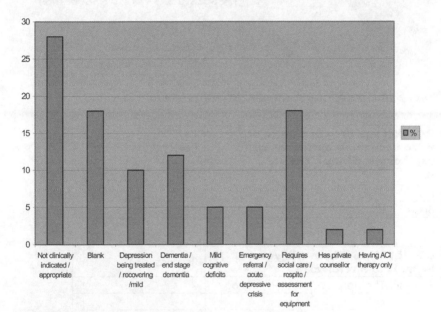

% of those not requiring psychological help

Q3. If YES, please tick ONE or MORE boxes which describe why help is needed:	Responses	%
Bereavement	2	3
Depression	14	19
Anxiety	12	17
Dementia	16	22
Neuropsychological	5	7
Assessment / Repeat Assessment	9	12
Memory Problems	14	19
Other: Cancer Phobia	1	1

Figure 13.3   Reasons for Psychological Help

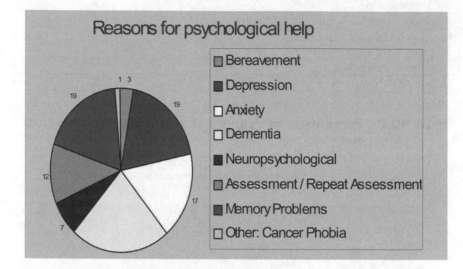

Note: Some people had more than one reason

Q4. Will you or your service or ward be making a referral for psychological help? YES/NO	Responses
Yes	10
No	36
Blank	22

Q5. If YES, to whom will you be making a referral?	Responses
Professor Thompson /Clinical Psychology	7
CPN service	2
Blank	59

Q6a. If NO, is this because there is no psychology service in your locality?	Responses
No psychology service provision	17
Refer to OT first	2
CPN support	2
Other	13
Blank	34

Q6b. If No, what will happen now?	Responses
OT assessment	2
GP care	2
CPN support	2
Blank	62

Analysis

28 patients were identified as requiring psychological help (Q1). 7 of them (25%) were to be referred to Clinical Psychology and 2 were to be referred to the CPN service (Q5). Hence, it would seem that patients were being considered for referral for psychological help. Therefore, the results of the audit fall within the guidelines of the NSF.

However, it is unclear from the data whether the remaining 40 patients were considered appropriately, as more sensitive information regarding individual circumstances was not included. Also, responses were to be confidential and anonymous.

Importantly, of the 36 'NO referral for psychological help' responses (Q4), 17 (47 %) were because there was no psychology service provision in Crawley and Horsham (Q6a). To date, this service is not funded.

Conclusions

There is a growing demand on clinical neuropsyhology services within the NHS. It is not just people who present with the signs of 'dementia' that require specialist services; however, this is a particularly needy group because there are often many associated problems including the considerable impact upon family, friends and carers.

Genetic Link with Dementia

Studies concerning the genetics of Alzheimer's disease, in particular, continue (for example, Cordell et al., 1995; Mann, 1995). The S182 gene located on chromosome 14 has been reported as being representative of the majority of early-onset, familial cases (Schellenberg, Bird & Wijsman, 1992).

Previously, mutations in the amyloid precursor protein (APP) gene located on chromosome 21 (see page 38) were reported as being implicated in later- onset, familial cases. Apolipoprotein E4 (a chromosome 19 gene) has been shown to be involved in late and spontancous forms of the disease (Poirier et al., 1993; Kuusisto, Kiovisto & Kervinen, 1994; Owen, Liddel & McGuffin, 1994; Lucotte, Turpin & Raisonnier, 1995), and another early form of Alzheimer's disease has been identified by Bird and Schellenberg (Bouthet, 1995) in a family kinship referred to as the 'Volga Germans'. Within this kinship, the chromosome 14 and 21 gene mutations were excluded, yet a gene with a similar sequence to that of the S182 gene was isolated from a gene library and found to bear a sequence mutation in the Volga German families (Bouthet, 1995).

A study of Alzheimer's disease in Finland has revealed a significantly higher incidence in monozygotic twins than in dizygotic twins. The finding supports the hypothesis that genetic factors contribute to the cause of Alzheimer's disease. In contrast, the incidence of vascular and mixed dementia was no different between monozygotic and dizygotic individuals (Räihä et al., 1996). However, the researchers comment that although their results confirm the involvement of a genetic component in Alzheimer's disease, they still believe there is a need to identify environmental triggers, because the age of onset was identical in only two pairs, and varied by as much as 15 years in the rest. Indeed, a similar conclusion has been reached in earlier studies (for example, Van Duijn, Clayton & Chandra, 1994). Longitudinal studies are very important for investigating environmental effects and also general risk factors in senile dementia (Sluss, Gruenberg & Kramer, 1981).

Medical Treatment for Alzheimer's Disease

In a study by Aarsland, Cummings and Kaufer (1995), 37 patients consecutively admitted to an outpatient clinic and diagnosed as having possible or probable Alzheimer's disease were routinely tested and medically examined. A fixed dose-titration schedule of tacrine (tetrahydroaminoacridine) was employed, the initial dose being 40 mg/day. Subsequently, the daily dose was increased by 40 mg every sixth week, until side-effects or a dose of 160 mg/day was achieved. Alanine aminotransferase (ALAT) levels were monitored weekly; dose escalation continued only in the presence of acceptable ALAT levels.

The principal finding in this study was that nine Alzheimer's disease patients (24 per cent) achieved the predetermined criterion for being a responder to tacrine treatment. This is comparable to the response rate in other studies. Eagger, Levy and Sahakian (1991) also reported dose-related improvement in cognitive functioning after treatment with tacrine in their large-scale study. However, Aarsland, Cummings and Kaufer (1995) advise caution in interpreting results, as the high attrition rate of their patients was due to increasing ALAT. Only 10 of the 37 patients (27 per cent) completed the scheduled dose-titration to 160 mg. However, 8 of the 9 responders improved on

40 mg or 80 mg, suggesting that increasing the tacrine dose above 80 mg does not contribute significantly to the response rate.

Few studies have focused on which mental functions respond to treatment with cholinergic drugs in Alzheimer's disease patients. It is known that cholinergic activity is important for learning and memory (Collerton, 1986) as well as for language, and that anticholinergic drugs induce sedation. The improved cognitive functioning on acetylcholinesterase inhibitors may be mediated through an effect on alertness and attentional function (Aarsland, Cummings & Kaufer, 1995).

Redefining Dementia

In Morris's (1994b) comprehensive paper on recent developments in the neuropsychology of dementia, he questions the simplicity of Lishman's (1987) definition of dementia: 'an acquired global impairment of intellect, memory and personality'. Morris (1994b) suggests that this definition:

> obscures the main outcome of recent research, which is that: (1) not all cognitive processes are impaired, at least in the early stages; (2) those processes that are more severely impaired can be related to the underlying neurobiological changes. In other words, the profile of different dementias is not random, but can be linked to damage to different areas of the brain or neurochemical systems; and (3) knowledge of preserved versus impaired functioning can yield important diagnostic information, as well as suggesting strategies for management and rehabilitation (p. 85).

Dementia has been the subject of vigorous investigation over the years (for example, Morris & Fulling, 1988; Lambert & Bieliauskas, 1993; Morris, 1994b), particularly with regard to how changes in neuropathology lead to sometimes subtle changes in clinical presentations. For example, in a study of 113 patients, Steingart et al. (1987) found that patients with leuko-araiosis (patchy or diffuse lucencies in the white matter) had significantly lower mean scores on the Extended Scale for Dementia.

The presence of neurofibrillary tangles and senile plaques has already been shown to be indicative of dementia (Crystal et al., 1988) with patients showing typical clinical changes in immediate memory, personality (for example, becoming socially withdrawn) and disorientation, highlighted by standardised neuropsychological tests such as the WMS-R (Wechsler, 1981b), the Beck Depression Inventory (Beck & Steer, 1987) and Mini-Mental State Examination (Folstein, Folstein & McHugh, 1975), respectively. Of course, such tools are only useful when accompanying a thorough clinical interview, which is always helpful if facts can be corroborated with a near relative or close friend of the patient being examined.

Callosal atrophy has been shown to be significantly related to the total and verbal IQs of the Wechsler Adult Intelligence Scale for patients with Alzheimer's disease (Yamauchi et al., 1993), and localisation of lesions in Korsakoff's syndrome has been linked with performance differences in patients on the Peterson short-term memory task and Wisconsin card sort test (Mayes et al., 1988). Neuropsychological examination has also yielded clinically helpful results in the study and identification of frontal lobe dementia (Royall & Mahurin, 1994), where two bedside measures (the Executive Interview and the Qualitative Evaluation of Dementia) have been developed to classify patients. Others (for example, Kumar & Gottlieb, 1993) argue that this newly-emerging syndrome should be termed 'frontotemporal dementia' because of the functional implication of both temporal and frontal regions of the brain.

Many clinicians consider that the inability to recall information or events over a period of minutes, days or weeks is a hallmark of dementia, particularly Alzheimer's disease (Morris, 1994b). This type of memory has been termed 'episodic' memory, to distinguish it from semantic memory (knowledge about the world, including rules, concepts and facts) (see page 47 and Tulving, 1983). Morris (1994b) and Morris and Kopelman (1986) view the episodic memory deficit in Alzheimer's disease as an amnesic syndrome overlayed by various processing deficits, which in turn contribute to memory impairment. Many Alzheimer's disease patients display the classical, pure amnesic syndrome, which outstrips other cognitive impairments in terms of severity, but is complicated by processing deficits, such as the language and visuospatial impairments associated with Alzheimer's disease.

Morris (1994b) suggests that the 'main' memory deficit appears to relate directly to damage in the mesiotemporal lobe, including the hippocampus (Esiri, 1991). The role of the hippocampal formation in memory has long been established, with damage relating to memory resulting from a variety of causes, including mesiotemporal lobe sclerosis and ischaemia (Parkin, 1991; Squire, 1992).

Autobiographical memories also appear to be affected in Alzheimer's disease: a common clinical impression is that recent memories are poorly remembered, but memories for the distant past are relatively preserved (Morris, 1994b). These distant memories, termed 'remote memory' (Kopelman, 1989), extend over periods of years rather than days or weeks. However, there is mounting evidence to suggest that the deficit in remote memory is also impaired for both recent and distant memories. Sagar et al. (1984) investigated remote memory in Alzheimer's disease patients using the Famous Faces Test (Albert, Butters & Levin, 1979). Their patients showed impairment for both well-known and less well-known faces and the deficit was relatively constant across the time period.

Attentional impairments have frequently been reported in patients with Alzheimer's disease (Mattis, 1988b). However, there have been varying uses of the term 'attention'. One meaning refers to maintaining a state of alertness or vigilance, the degree of receptiveness to external stimuli (Allport, 1989), for example, when monitoring a visual display for long periods. A second meaning, 'selective attention', is the facility to shift attention between different external stimuli, such as the ability to scan and fixate individual faces in a crowd (Humphreys & Bruce, 1989) or the ability to 'tune into' one particular conversation at a cocktail party (Morris, 1994b). A third meaning, 'divided attention', is when attention may be split equally or almost simultaneously between different stimuli.

Morris (1994b) concludes that 'dementia' is a multifaceted disorder and treatment and management should capitalise on preserved functioning. It is known that Alzheimer's disease patients cope much better when their attention is not divided; cueing helps both encoding and retrieval in episodic memory, and memory re-training programmes, such as reality orientation (Miller & Morris, 1993), can substantially help dementing patients. There is growing optimism about gaining better understanding of the complexities of the various different types of dementia, with ever-advancing technologies such as neuro-imaging and neuropsychological testing.

There have been many changes over the years in the way we have both treated and managed dementia. As our knowledge of the validity and reliability of screening tests for the early detection of dementia advances, perhaps our approach to managing dementia might change. One fact is certain: the population of older people is increasing; therefore, we should strive to deliver better health and social services with the aim of ultimately providing a better lifestyle for people diagnosed as 'living with' rather than 'suffering from' dementia.

Further Reading

Aarsland, D., Cummings, J.L. & Kaufer, D. (1995), 'Tacrine in Alzheimer's disease: Which patients and which mental functions improve?' *Alzheimer's Research*, 1, 3: 133–6.

Alberoni, M., Baddeley, A.D., Della Sala, S. & Logic, R. (1992), 'Keeping track of a conversation: Impairments in Alzheimer's disease',

International Journal of Geriatric Psychiatry, 7: 639–46.

Davies, S. (1996), 'Neuropsychological assessment of the older person', in Woods, R.T. (ed.), *Clinical Psychology of Ageing*, Chichester: John Wiley.

Fromholt, P. & Larsen, S.F. (1991), 'Autobiographical memory in normal aging and primary degenerative dementia (dementia of Alzheimer type)', *Journal of Gerontology (Psychological Sciences)*, 46, 3: 85–91.

Kapur, N.K., Thompson, S.B.N., Cook, P., Lang, D., et al. (1996), 'Anterograde but not retrograde memory loss following combined mammillary body and medial thalamic lesions', *Neuropsycholologia*, 34, 1: 1-8.

Leuchter, A.F., Newton, T.F., Cook, I.A., Walter, D.O., et al. (1992), 'Changes in brain functional connectivity in Alzheimer-type and multi-infarct dementia', *Brain*, 115, 1,543–61.

Morris, R.G. (1994b), 'Recent developments in the neuropsychology of dementia', *International Review of Psychiatry*, 6: 85–107.

Morris, R.G. & McKiernan, F. (1993), 'Neuropsychological investigation of dementia', in Burns, A. & Levy, R. (eds), *Dementia*, London: Chapman & Hall.

Morris, R.G., Wheatley, J. & Britton, P.G. (1983), 'Retrieval from long-term memory in senile dementia: Cued recall revisited', *British Journal of Clinical Psychology*, 22: 141–2.

Tuokko, H. & Crockett, D. (1989), 'Cued recall and memory disorders in dementia', *Journal of Clinical & Experimental Neuropsychology*, 11: 278-294.

Test Your Long-term Memory

The following questions have been compiled as a "rough-and-ready" test of your general knowledge. They are intended to test your memory for past events and have been divided into six decades (ie *1940s, 1950s, 1960s, 1970s, 1980s, 1990s)* according to the age of the person being tested. For example, someone born in the *1920s is* more likely to know the answers to questions from the *1940s* onwards than someone born later in the *1950s.* However, you may wish to test yourself on all of the questions or they may be read out to someone else mixing up the different decades.

In Section 1, there are six questions (except for the 1940s where there are 10) each with a choice of three statements: A, B or C. Choose the correct statement and then answer the supplementary question asked in Section 2. All answers are provided in Section 3.

Please note that this is in no way a definitive test of your memory but serves to act as a guide to memory functioning and may indicate *broadly* whether or not the person being tested is starting to forget events that *they used to* remember well.

Section 1: Choice of Statements

1940s

Q1.
A Ninety German bombers are shot down over Russia.
B Ninety German bombers are shot down over Britain.
C Ninety German bombers are shot down over Poland.

Q2.
A The liner, Empress of Britain, is sunk.
B The floating hotel, Empress of Britain, is sunk.
C The warship, Empress of Britain, is sunk.

Q3.
A The blockade of Berlin by Poland is lifted.
B The blockade of Berlin by the USSR is lifted.
C The blockade of Berlin by Britain is lifted.

Q4.

A NATO Treaty signed in Hong Kong.

B NATO Treaty signed in London.

C NATO Treaty signed in Washington.

Q5.

A USSR stops road and rail communication between Berlin and the West.

B USSR stops road and rail communication between Munich and the East.

C USSR stops road and rail communication between Warsaw and the West.

Q6.

A Bread rationing in America because of world shortage of wheat.

B Bread rationing in Britain because of world shortage of wheat.

C Bread rationing in Eire becaues of world shortage of wheat.

Q7.

A Big Ben is destroyed during heavy bombing.

B House of Commons is destroyed during heavy bombing.

C Trafalgar Square is destroyed during heavy bombing.

Q8.

A Malta is awarded the Victoria Cross.

B Malta is awarded the Iron Cross.

C Malta is awarded the George Cross.

Q9.

A Japanese invade Burma.

B Chinese invade Burma.

C Allied troops invade Burma.

Q10.

A British waterways are nationalised.

B British parks are nationalised.

C British railways are nationalised.

1950s

Q1.

A Underground fire during tunnelling at Dartford kills 80 workmen.

B Sides of quarry collapse in Lincoln killing 80 quarrymen.

C Undergraound disaster in a colliery at Cresswell kills 80 miners.

Q2.

A Experiments revealed the skull of the `Piltdown Man' to be a
    primitive ancestor of the human race.

B Experiments revealed the skull of the `Piltdown Man' to be a forty
    year old hoax.

C Experiments revealed the skull of the `Piltdown Man' to be the
    relative of a later archaeological finding.

Q3.

A Britain's first hydrogen bomb is dropped on Christmas Island.

B Britain's first nuclear submarine docks at Christmas Island.

C Britain's first bouncing bomb is dropped on Christmas Island.

Q4.

A Army seige Panmunjon starting Korean war.

B Armistice signed at Panmunjon to end Korean war.

C Vietnamese take Panmunjon in Korean war.

Q5.

A Princess Elizabeth returns from abroad after hearing about riding
    accident.

B Princess Elizabeth returns from abroad after hearing about car
    crash.

C Princess Elizabeth returns from abroad after hearing about death
    of her father.

Q6.

A Roger Bannister breaks four-minute mile.

B Roger Bannister breaks high-jump record.

C Roger Bannister breaks long-jump record.

1960s

Q1.

A A toxic leak from the tanker River Valley causes pollution in the
    River Exe.

B An oil spill from the tanker Tory Canyon causes pollution in the
    English Channel.

C A chemical spillage from the tanker Gulf Breeze causes pollution
    in the Irish Sea.

Q2.

A Israel and Egypt fight six-day war.

B Libya and Iraq fight six-day war.

C Uganda and Kenya fight six-day war.

Q3.
A US President orders Russia to remove missile sites from Cuba.
B Soviet President orders China to remove missile sites from
   Stalingrad.
C German Premier orders Russia to remove missle sites from
   Eastern Germany.

Q4.
A Russian spacecraft with two cosmonauts lands on moon.
B Chinese satellite with two monkeys lands on moon.
C American spacecraft with two astronauts lands on moon.

Q5.
A The Beatles receive a major honour by Queen for their services to
   music.
B The Beatles honour the Queen in a remembrance concert.
C The Beatles receive an award from the US President

Q6.
A Archbishop Makarios returns to Cyprus after being deported from
   another country.
B Reverend Makinos leaves Cyprus for another country.
C Archbishop Makarios returns to Syria after being deported from
   another country.

1970s

Q1.
A In Honduras, 200 bodies are found, all believed to have been shot
   by mistake by terrorists.
B In New Guinea, 541 bodies of members of the newly formed
   government are found, all believed to have been murdered.
C In Guyana, 912 bodies of members of the People's Temple are
   found, all believed to have committed suicide.

Q2.
A Kenya makes a unilateral declaration of Independence.
B Rhodesia makes a unilateral declaration of Independence.
C Zambia makes a unilateral declaration of Independence.

Q3.

A Twelve IRA gunmen are cornered by police in a basement seige in Haze Street, Brighton.

B Two IRA gunmen are arrested in a seige in Balmoral Castle, Scotland.

C Four IRA gunmen are surrounded by police in a seige in Balcombe Street, London.

Q4.

A Ayatollah Khomeini returns to Afganistan after many years in power.

B Ayatollah Khomeini returns to Iraq after many years abroad.

C Ayatollah Khomeini makes a triumphant return to Iran after many years in exile.

Q5.

A Chi-Chi dies in London zoo.

B Ciao-Ciao has baby in Chessington zoo.

C Ping-Ping survives operation in Jersey zoo.

Q6.

A Cut-price air fares announced by Rupert Murdoch, between Hong Kong and New York.

B Cut-price skybus air service, run by Clive Sinclair,

C Cut-price skytrain air service, run by Freddie Laker, starts between London and New York.

1980s

Q1.

A Eleven killed and sixty people are injured by an IRA bomb attack on Remembrance Day in Northern Ireland.

B Twelve killed and thirty people are injured by an IRA attack on Orangeman's Day in Northern Ireland.

C Eleven killed and twenty people are injured by an IRA attack on St Patrick's Day in Northern Ireland.

Q2.

A Britain fights Falklands War.

B Britain fights Hong Kong War.

C Britain fights Gibraltar War.

Q3.
A Airliner crashes on London bridge after wing fails.
B Airliner crashes on British motorway after engine catches fire
C Airliner crashes on British football pitch after door falls off.

Q4.
A Arsonist sets fire to old people's home in Sussex town killing 21 OAPs.
B IRA bomb in Wiltshire town kills 16 soldiers in pub.
C Lone gunman shoots dead 14 people in Berkshire town.

Q5.
A Soviet Union accidently shoots down Korean aircraft that enters its air space.
B Czechoslovakia accidentally shoots down Russian aircraft that enters its air space.
C Poland accidentally shoots down German aircraft that enters its air space.

Q6.
A Yacht with French passengers capsizes and sinks in Italian port with 20 dead.
B Ferry with British passengers rolls over and sinks in Belgian port with 200 dead.
C Cruiseliner with German passengers keels over and sinks in Dutch port with 300 dead.

1990s

Q1.
A Air France jumbo jet crashes into Paris hotel.
B British Airways jet crashes into control tower in New York.
C El Al cargo jet crashes into block of flats.

Q2.
A IRA bomb explodes in Welsh town killing three pensioners out shopping.
B IRA bomb explodes in Lancashire town killing two boys out shopping.
C IRA bomb explodes in Sussex sports centre killing six youths.

Q3.
A Grand National horse race abandoned after flooding.
B Grand National horse race abandoned after false start.

C Grand National horse race abandoned after Animal Rights' protest.

Q4.
A Czech parliament taken over by army after invasion by Soviets.
B Polish parliament falls after Czechs move in.
C Soviet parliament stormed by army after dissident MPs take over building.

Q5.
A IRA launch mortar bomb attack on 10 Downing Street.
B IRA use tear gas to invade House of Commons.
C IRA plant bomb inside Buckingham Palace.

Q6.
A Japan conducts underwater nuclear tests despite European bans.
B India conducts underwater nuclear tests despite European disapproval.
C China conducts airborne nuclear tests despite World-wide disapproval.

2000s

Q1.
A Olympics is held in Norway.
B Olympics is held in Athens.
C Olympics is held in Portugal.

Q2.
A Labour elected to govern Britain.
B Conservatives elected to govern Britain.
C Liberals elected to govern Britain.

Q3.
A Vehicle registration "51" denotes month registered.
B Vehicle registration "51" denotes year registered.
C Vehicle registration "51" denotes month and year registered.

Q4.
A The new Queen Margaret is launched.
B The new Queen Mary is launched.
C The new Queen Mary III is launched.

Q5.
A Mark won Channel 5's 'Little Brother'.
B Angela won ITV's 'Big Sister'.
C Anthony won Channel 4's 'Big Brother'.

Q6.
A Russians trapped in small submarine are saved.
B Polish trapped in small satellite die.
C Czechs save Russians in small ship.

Section 2: Supplementary Questions

For each question, firstly, give the correct month (if possible) and the year.

1940s

1. What was significant about *these* types of raids?
2. Which country sunk the ship?
3. Who was the President of Russia?
4. What was the name given to this Treaty?
5. What was `Operation Carter Paterson'?
6. What other commodity was also running short?
7. What did MPs use as a temporary building?
8. Why was Malta awarded this honour?
9. Which city in Burma was evacuated?
10. What is `nationalisation'?

1950s

1. What caused the disaster?
2. In which county was the `Piltdown Man' found?
3. Where is Christmas Island?
4. How long did the war last?
5. From which country did she return?
6. What nationality is Roger Bannister?

1960s

1. How was the oil stopped?
2. Who won?
3. What happened next?
4. What was the name of the first man on the moon?

5. What award did they receive?
6. What country was he deported to?

1970s

1. How did they commit suicide?
2. Who was the Prime Minister of Rhodesia?
3. What was the outcome?
4. In which city and country was he in exile?
5. What species of animal was Chi-Chi?
6. Was it successful?

1980s

1. In which town did this happen?
2. Who was the war against?
3. Where did this happen?
4. What was the name of the town?
5. Was it a military jet or a passenger jet?
6. What was the name of the ship?

1990s

1. In which European city did this happen?
2. What was the name of the town?
3. Was the race re-run?
4. Who was the President at the time?
5. Was the Cabinet meeting at that time?
6. What country followed with the same tests?

2000s

1. Was the Winter Olympics held in the same city?
2. Who is the new Prime Minister?
3. How many times in the year does the new registration change?
4. Where was the destination of its maiden voyage?
5. What town is the winner from?
6. Which country's navy save them?

Section 3: Answers

Answers are given in this order: A/B/C; month & year; supplementary answer.

1940s

1. B; Jul. 1940; First daylight raids by Germans.
2. A; Oct. 1940; Germany.
3. B; May 1949; Stalin.
4. C; Apr. 1949; North Atlantic Treaty.
5. A; Jun. 1948; Food supplies dropped by allied pilots.
6. B; Jul. 1946; Coal.
7. B; May 1941; House of Lords.
8. C; Apr. 1942; Suffered sustained bombing by Germans in World War II.
9. A; Jan. 1942; Rangoon.
10. C: Jan. 1948; Public ownership of companies and government accountability.

1950s

1. C; Sep. 1950; Conveyor belt began burning which set fire to electric cables.
2. B; Nov. 1953; East Sussex.
3. A; May 1957; Central Pacific.
4. B; Jul. 1953; Three years.
5. C; Feb. 1952; Kenya.
6. A; May 1954; British.

1960s

1. B; Mar. 1967; Oil slick bombed to sink tanker and burn off oil.
2. A; Jun. 1967; Israel.
3. A; Oct. 1962; Americans created naval blockade resulting in Soviets dismantling missile sites.
4. C; Jul. 1969; Neil Armstrong.
5. A; Dec. 1965; MBE.
6. A; Aug. 1960; Seychelles.

1970s

1. C; Nov. 1978; Drank cyanide.
2. B; Mar. 1970; Ian Smith.

3. C; Dec. 1975; Hostages released and gunmen surrendered.
4. C; Feb. 1979; Paris, France.
5. A (very sad); May 1972; Giant Panda.
6. C; Sep. 1977; No.

1980s

1. A; Nov. 1987; Enniskillen.
2. A; Apr.-Jun. 1982; Argentina.
3. B; Jan. 1989; Kegworth, Leicestershire.
4. C; Aug. 1987; Hungerford.
5. A; Sep. 1983; Passenger jet.
6. B; Mar. 1987; Herald of Free Enetrprise.

1990s

1. C; Oct. 1992; Amsterdam.
2. B: 1993; Warrington.
3. B; Mar. 1993; No.
4. C; 1993; Boris Yeltsin.
5. A; Feb. 1991; Yes.
6. B; May 1998; Pakistan.

2000s

1. B; July 2004; No.
2. A; May 2005; Tony Blair.
3. C; Sep. 2001; Two.
4. B; Mar. 2003; New York.
5. C; Aug. 2005; Newcastle.
6. A; Aug. 2005; British.

Glossary of Terms

(Sources: Thompson & Morgan, 1996; Wainwright, Fergusson & Martin, 1984.)

ablation Surgical removal of tissue, a part of the body, or an abnormal growth, usually by cutting.

abulia Absence or impairment of will-power, commonly a symptom of schizophrenia.

acetylcholine Acetic acid ester of the organic base choline: the neurotransmitter released at the synapses of parasympathetic nerves and at neuromuscular junctions. *See* cholinesterase.

aetiology Science of the causes of disease.

agnosia Disorder of the brain whereby the patient cannot interpret sensations correctly, although the sense organs and nerves conducting sensation to the brain are functioning normally.

allele (allelomorph) One or two or more alternative forms of a gene, only one of which can be present in a chromosome.

amyloid deposits A glycoprotein, resembling starch, that is deposited in the internal organs in amyloidosis.

amyloidogenic gene Gene responsible for producing amyloid protein.

(amyloid) precursor protein Protein used to produce another in the series.

amyotrophy A progressive loss of muscle bulk associated with weakness, caused by disease of the nerve that supplies the affected muscle.

anoxia Condition in which the tissues of the body receive inadequate amounts of oxygen.

anterior horn cell inclusion Front outgrowth structure of the brain. (See an anatomy textbook for details of function.)

anxiolytic Usually refers to a drug which aims to reduce levels of anxiety.

aphasia Disorder of language affecting the generation of speech and its understanding. It is caused by disease in the left half of the brain (the dominant hemisphere) in a right-handed person.

apraxia Inability to make skilled movements with accuracy. This is a disorder of the cerebral cortex most often caused by disease of the parietal lobes of the brain.

arteriosclerosis Any of several conditions affecting the arteries, such as atherosclerosis; Mönckeberg's degeneration, in which calcium is deposited in the arteries as part of the ageing process; and arteriolarsclerosis, in which the walls of small arteries become thickened due to ageing or hypertension.

articulatory loop system System thought to be responsible in theories of memory functioning.

articulatory rehearsal mechanism *See* articulatory loop system.

astrocystosis Production of any brain tumour derived from non-nervous supporting cells (glia), which may be benign or malignant. In adults astrocytomas are usually found in the cerebral hemispheres but in children they also occur in the cerebellum.

autosomal dominant gene A chromosome that is not a sex chromosome which occurs in pairs in diploid cells. Dominant refers to that gene taking preference usually during replication or division.

basal ganglia Several large masses of grey matter embedded deep within the white matter of the cerebrum. They include the caudate and lenticular nuclei (together known as the corpus striatum) and the amygdaloid nucleus. The lenticular nucleus consists of the putamen and globus pallidus. The basal ganglia are involved with the regulation of voluntary movements at a subconscious level.

brain stem The enlarged extension upwards within the sull of the spinal cord, consisting of the medulla oblongata, the pons, and the midbrain.

callosal atrophy Degeneration (wastage) of the corpus callosum.

caseness Falls into the category associated with a clinical disorder or symptom, for example, caseness depression – clinical depression.

centrimorgan Minute measurement used in genetics for comparing relative size of genes.

cerebellum The largest part of the hindbrain, bulging back behind the pons and the medulla oblongata and overhung by the occipital lobes of the cerebrum. The cerebellum is essential for the maintenance of muscle tone, balance, and the synchronization of activity in groups of muscles under voluntary control, converting muscular contractions into smooth coordinated movement.

cerebral palsy Developmental abnormality of the brain resulting in weakness and incoordination of the limbs and often caused by injury during birth. The most common disability is a spastic paralysis which may slowly increase from contractures to cause fixed deformities of the limbs.

cholinergic Describing nerve fibres that release acetycholine as a neurotransmitter.

cholinesterase (inhibitor) An enzyme that breaks down a choline ester into its choline and acid components. The term usually refers to acetylcholinesterase, which breaks down the neurotransmitter acetylcholine into choline and acetic acid.

chorea A jerky involuntary movement particularly affecting the shoulders, hips, and face. The symptoms are due to disease of the basal ganglia. Huntington's chorea is an inherited form in which the involuntary movements are accompanied by a progressive dementia: there is widespread neuronal degeneration throughout the brain. Sydenham's chorea affects children and is associated with rheumatic fever. It responds to mild sedatives.

choreiform movements *See* chorea.

cognitive abulia *See* abulia.

confabulation Invention of circumstantial but fictitious detail about events supposed to have occurred in the past. Usually this is to disguise a loss of memory; it typically occurs in Korsakoff's syndrome.

CT (computerised [axial] tomography) Technique of neuroimaging using a computer to provide an integrated three-dimensional image of the soft structures of the body, particularly the brain. It can reveal the presence of tumours, fluid, etc.

declarative memory Often associated with skills and routines, for example, knowing how the engine works in a car is considered to be the responsibility of declarative memory.

demyelination A disease process selectively damaging the myelin sheaths in the central or peripheral nervous system. Demyelination may be the primary disorder in multiple sclerosis, or it may occur after head injury or strokes.

difference score Score after subtracting one score from another. The result may be positive, negative or without a sign (absolute score).

dizygotic twins Also known as fraternal twins. Twins resulting from the simultaneous fertilisation of two eggs; they may be of different sexes and are no more alike than ordinary siblings.

dyscalculia Inability to calculate, for example, arithmetic.

dysphagia Difficulty or disorder in swallowing.

dysphasia *See* aphasia. 'Dys' versus 'a' usually refers to partial versus complete absence of disorder of language affecting generation of speech.

EEG Electroencephalogram is a tracing produced from converting the electrical activity recorded from different parts of the brain using a machine known as an electroencephalograph. The technique, electroencephalography, is used to detect and locate structural disease, such as tumours, in the brain; it is also used in the diagnosis and management of epilepsy.

epidemiology Cause, prevalence and distribution of a disease.

episodic memory Memories for particular events, for example, knowing what you had for breafast.

extrapyramidal system System of nerve tracts and pathways connecting the cerebral cortex, basal ganglia, thalamus, cerebellum, reticular formation, and spinal neurones in complex circuits not included in the pyramidal system. It is mainly concerned with the regulation of stereotyped reflex muscular movements.

functional MRI Magnetic resonance imaging (MRI) is particularly useful for plotting cerebral blood flow and for analysing lesions in the brain. It uses a large rotating magnet creating a strong magnetic field around the patient's head. An image of the head and brain is created by summing 'pictures' taken at different time intervals.

hippocampus A swelling in the floor of the lateral ventricle of the brain. It contains complex foldings of cortical tissue and is involved in the workings of the limbic system.

hydrocephalus An abnormal increase in the amount of cerebrospinal fluid within the ventricles of the brain. In childhood, before the sutures of the skull have fused, hydrocephalus makes the head enlarge. In adults, it raises the intracranial pressure with consequent drowsiness and vomiting. Spina bifida is commonly associated with hydrocephalus.

hypermetamorphosis Tendency to react by exploring environmental stimuli as soon as they are noticed.

hyperoxygenation Too much oxygen in the blood. *See* hyperventilation.

hyperventilation Breathing at an abnormally rapid rate at rest. This causes unconsciousness by lowering carbon dioxide concentration in the blood.

hypomania A mild degree of mania. Elated mood leads to faulty judgement; behaviour lacks the usual social restraints and the sexual drive is increased; speech is rapid and animated; the individual is energetic but not persistent and tends to be irritable.

hysterical Describing a symptom that is not due to organic disease, is produced unconsciously, and from which the individual derives some gain. It can also describe a kind of personality disorder characterised by instability and shallowness of feelings.

idiopathic Denoting a disease or condition the cause of which is not known or that arises spontaneously.

infarct A small localised area of dead tissue produced as a result of an inadequate blood supply.

ischaemia An inadequate flow of blood to a part of the body, caused by constriction or blockage of the blood vessels supplying it.

Kernig's sign Symptom of meningitis in which the patient is unable to extend his legs at the knee when the thighs are held at a right angle to the body. (V. Kernig (1840–1917), Russian physician).

limbic system A complex system of nerve pathways and networks in the brain that is involved in the expression of instinct and mood in activities of the endocrine and motor systems of the body. Among the brain regions involved are the amygdala, hippocampal formation, and hypothalamus.

magnetic resonance imaging *See* functional MRI.

meningitis Inflammation of the meninges due to viral or bacterial infection. Meningitis causes an intense headache, fever, loss of appetite, intolerance to light and sound, rigidity of muscles, especially those in the neck (*see* Kernig's sign), and in severe cases convulsions, vomiting, and delirium leading to death. Bacterial meningitis can be effectively treated with antibiotics or sulphonamides.

monozygotic twins Also known as identical twins. Resulting from the fertilisation of a single egg cell that subsequently divides to give two separate features. They are of the same sex and otherwise genetically identical.

multi-infarcts A number of small localised areas of dead tissue produced as a result of an inadequate blood supply. Multi-infarct dementia (old term, now 'Vascular dementia'): dementia resulting from multi-infarcts in the brain versus arteriosclerotic or parenchymatous dementia.

myoclonus A sudden spasm of the muscles typically lifting and flexing the arms. Myoclonus is a major feature of some progressive neurological illnesses with extensive degeneration of brain cells.

neurasthenia A set of psychological and physical symptoms, including fatigue, irritability, headache, and dizziness. It can be caused by organic damage, such as a head injury, or it can be due to neurosis.

neuroleptic Any drug that induces an altered state of consciousness, such as a major tranquilliser.

neurotransmitter A chemical substance, such as acetylcholine, released from nerve endings to transmit impulses across synapses to other nerves and across the minute gaps between the nerves and the muscles or glands that they supply.

normative Establishing a norm; data that cannot be ordered, for example, labels or names of items.

nosology Classification of diseases.

optic neuritis Also known as retrobulbar neuritis, it is the inflammation of the optic nerve behind the eye, causing increasingly blurred vision. Optic neuritis is one of the symptoms of multiple sclerosis but it can also occur as an isolated lesion.

paresis Muscular weakness caused by disease of the nervous system. It implies a lesser degree of weakness than paralysis, although the two words are often used interchangeably.

perseveration Excessive persistence at a task that prevents the individual from turning his/her attention to new situations. It is a symptom of organic disease of the brain and sometimes of obsessive neurosis.

PET (photon emission tomography) Elaboration of the CT scan method of neuroimaging where a radioactive isotope label is injected intravenously in order to monitor cerebral blood flow (by blood glucose metabolising) during irradiation.

phenylketonuria Inborn defect of protein metabolism causing an excess of the amino acid phenylalanine in the blood, which damages the nervous system and leads to severe mental retardation. The gene responsible for phenylketonuria is recessive, so that a child is affected only if both parents are carriers of the defective gene.

prodromal Relating to the period of time between the appearance of the first symptoms of an infectious disease and the development of a rash or fever.

psychogenic Of psychological rather than organic origin.

rubella or German measles Highly contagious virus infection, mainly occurring in childhood. Symptoms include headache, sore throat, and slight fever, followed by swelling and soreness of the neck and erruption of a rash of minute pink spots, spreading from the face and neck to the rest of the body. Rubella can cause foetal malformations during early pregnancy.

septum A partition or dividing wall within a structure.

SPET (single photon emission tomography) *See* PET.

standard deviation Statistical term representing the proximity of data to the norm.

stenosis Abnormal narrowing of a passage or opening, such as a blood vessel or heart valve. (Associated terms: aortic stenosis, mitral stenosis, pyloric stenosis.)

(subdural) haematoma An accumulation of blood within the tissues that clots to form a solid swelling. Injury, disease of the blood vessels, or a clotting disorder of the blood are the usual causative factors. Subdural haematoma is caused by tearing of the veins where they cross the space beneath the dura of the brain.

transient ischaemic attack Stroke which is usually not life-threatening and may consist of a series of small strokes which may result from an inadequate flow of blood to the brain. Associated term: ischaemia.

trisomy A condition in which there is one extra chromosome present in each cell in addition to the normal (diploid) chromosome set. The cause of such disorders as Down's syndrome.

uncus Any hooked-shaped structure, especially a projection of the lower surface of the cerebral hemisphere.

white matter Nerve tissue of the central nervous system that is paler in colour than the associated grey matter because it contains more nerve fibres and thus larger amounts of myelin.

Useful Journals and Magazines

Ageing
Alzheimer's Research
British Journal of Clinical Psychology
British Journal of Developmental Disabilities
British Journal of Occupational Therapy
British Journal of Therapy and Rehabilitation
British Medical
Journal of Community Care
European Journal of Neurology
The Journal of Cognitive Rehabilitation
Journal of Gerontology
Journal of Neurology, Neurosurgery and Psychiatry
The Lancet
Memory
Neuropsychologia

Bibliography

Aarsland, D., Cummings, J.L. & Kaufer, D. (1995), 'Tacrine in Alzheimer's disease: Which patients and which mental functions improve?', *Alzheimer's Research*, 1, 3: 133–6.

Acorn, S. & Andersen, S. (1990), 'Depression in multiple sclerosis: Critique of the research literature', *Journal of Neuroscience Nursing*, 22, 4: 209–14.

Agbayewa, M.D., Weir, J., Tuokko, H. & Beattie, L. (1991), 'Depression in dementia: Its impact on functional ability', *Dementia*, 2: 212–17.

Alberoni, M., Baddeley, A.D., Della Sala, S. & Logie, R. (1992), 'Keeping track of a conversation: Impairments in Alzheimer's disease', *International Journal of Geriatric Psychiatry*, 7: 639–46.

Albert, M.L. (1978), 'Subcortical Dementia', in Katzman, R., Terry, R.D. & Bick, K.L. (eds), *Alzheimer's Disease: Senile Dementia and Related Disorders*, New York: Raven Press.

Albert, M.S., Butters, N. & Levin, J. (1979), 'Temporal gradients in the retrograde amnesia of patients with alcoholic Korsakoff's disease', *Archives of Neurology*, 36: 211–16.

Alcott, D. (1993), 'Normal aging', in Stokes, G. & Goudie, F. (eds), *Working with Dementia*, Oxford: Winslow Press.

All Wales Specialist Nurse Group (1992), *A Statement for the Future: Mental Handicap Nursing in Wales*, Cardiff: Welsh Office.

Allen, P.A., Smith, A.F., Jerge, K.A. & Vires-Collins, H. (1997), 'Age differences in mental multiplication: Evidence for peripheral but not central decrements', *Journal of Gerontology*, 52; 2: P81-P90.

Allport, A. (1989), 'Visual Attention', in Posner, M.I. (ed.), *Foundations of Cognitive Science*, Cambridge, Massachusetts, MIT Press.

Alter, M., Neugut, R. & Kahana, E. (1978), 'Familial aggregates of Creutzfeldt-Jakob disease', *Neurology*, 28: 353.

APA (American Psychiatric Association) (1987), *Diagnostic and Statistical Manual of Mental Disorders – Revised (DSM-III-R)*. (3rd edn), Washington, DC: APA, 78–80.

APA (American Psychiatric Association) (1994), *Diagnostic and Statistical Manual of Mental Disorders (DSM-IV)* (4th edn,) Washington, DC: APA, 139–43.

Asperger, H. (1944), 'Die "autistischen Psychopathen" im Kindesalter' ('"Autistic psychiopaths" at an early age'), *Archiv für Psychiatrie und Nervenkrankheiten*, 117: 76–136.

Asperger, H. (1968), 'Zur differentialdiagnose des kindlichen Autismus' ('Towards a differential diagnosis of child autism'), *Acta Paedopsychiatrica*, 35: 136–45.

Asperger, H. (1979), 'Problems of infantile autism', *Communication*, 13: 45–52.

Atkinson, L. (1991a), 'Mental retardation and WAIS-R difference scores', *Journal of Mental Deficiency Research*, 35: 537–42.

Atkinson, L. (1991b), 'On WAIS-R differences scores in the standardization sample', *Psychological Assessment: A Journal of Consulting & Clinical Psychology*, 3: 288–91.

Atkinson, R.C. & Shiffrin, R.M. (1968), 'Human memory: A proposed system and its control processes', in Spence, K. & Spence, J. (eds), *The Psychology of Learning & Motivation*, New York: Academic Press.

Baddeley, A.D. (1978), 'The trouble with levels: A re-examination of Craik and Lockhart's framework for memory research', *Psychological Review*, 85: 139–52.

Baddeley, A.D. (1986), *Working Memory*, Oxford: Oxford University Press.

Baddeley, A.D. (1992), 'Working memory', *Science*, 255: 556–9.

Baddeley, A.D. (1996), *Human Memory* (Revised edn), Hove: Psychology Press.

Baddeley, A.D., Bressi, S., Della Sala, S., Logie, R., et al. (1991), 'The decline of working memory in Alzheimer's disease', *Brain*, 114: 2,521–42.

Baddeley, A.D. & Hitch, G.J. (1974), 'Working memory', in Bower, G. (ed.), *Recent Advances in Learning and Motivation*, Vol. 3, London: Academic Press.

Baddeley, A.D., Logie, R., Bressi, S., Della Sala, S., et al. (1986), 'Dementia and working memory', *Quarterly Journal of Experimental Psychology*, 38A: 603–18.

Baddeley, A.D., Thomson, N. & Buchanan, M. (1975), 'Word length and the structure of short-term memory', *Journal of Verbal Learning and Verbal Behavior*, 14: 575–89.

Baddeley, A.D. & Warrington, E.K. (1970), 'Amnesia and the distinction between long- and short-term memory', *Journal of Verbal Learning and Verbal Behavior*, 9: 176–89.

Baddeley, A.D., Wilson, B.A. & Watts, F. (1995), *Handbook of Memory Disorders*, Chichester: John Wiley. Baldwin, R.C. & Byrne, E.J. (1989), 'Psychiatric aspects of Parkinson's disease: Dementia, depression and psychosis', *British Medical Journal*, 299: 3–4. Barbul, A. (1990), 'Immune aspects of wound repair', *Clinical Plastic Surgery*, 17: 433–42.

Baldwin, R. (eds) (2003) *Young People with Dementia: A Multidisciplinary*

Approach. London: Martin Dunitz.

Barette, J. & Marsden, C.D. (1979), 'Attitudes of families to some aspects of Huntington's chorea', *Psychological Medicine*, 9: 327–36.

Barr, O. (1990), 'Down's syndrome and Alzheimer's disease – what is the link?', *Professional Nurse*, June: 465–8.

Bayles, K.A. & Boone, D. (1982) 'The potential of language tasks for identifying senile dementia', *Journal of Speech & Hearing Disorders*, 47: 210–17.

Bayles, K.A. & Kaszniak, A. (1987), *Communication and Cognition in Normal Ageing and Dementia*, Philadelphia: Taylor & Francis.

Beck, A.T. & Steer, R.A. (1987), *Beck Depression Inventory: Manual*, San Antonio: Harcourt Brace Jovanovich.

Beck, A.T., Steer, R.A. & Brown, G.K. (1996) *BDI-II Manual*. San Antonio: The Psychological Corporation.

Becker, J.T. (1988), 'Working memory and secondary memory deficits in Alzheimer's disease', *Journal of Clinical & Experimental Neuropsychology*, 6: 739-753.

Benton, A.L. & Hamsher, K. de S. (1983) *Multilingual Aphasia Examination*. Iowa: AJA Associates.

Benton Sivan A. (1992) *Benton Visual retention Test 5th Ed Manual*. San Antonio: The Psychological Corporation.

Benedict, K.B. & Nacoste, D.B. (1990), 'Dementia and depression in the elderly: A framework for addressing difficulties in differential diagnosis', *Clinical Psychology Review*, 10: 513–37.

Bennett, G. & Kingston, P. (1993), *Elder Abuse: Concepts, Theories and Interventions*, London: Chapman & Hall.

Bennett, T., Dittmar, C. & Raubach, S. (1991), 'Multiple sclerosis: Cognitive deficits and rehabilitation strategies', *Cognitive Rehabilitation*, September/ October: 18–23.

Benton, A.L. (1977), 'Interactive effects of old age and brain disease on reaction time', *Archives of Neurology*, 34: 369–70.

Benton, A.L., Eslinger, P.J. & Damasio, A.R. (1981), 'Normative observations on neuropsychological test performances in old age', *Journal of Clinical Neuropsychology*, 3: 33–42.

Benton, A.L. & Spreen, O. (1961), 'Visual memory test: The simulation of mental incompetence', *Archives of General Psychiatry*, 4; 79–83.

Benton, A.L. (1977), 'Interactive effects of old age and brain disease on reaction time', *Archives of Neurology, 34;* 369-370.

Benton, A.L. & Spreen, O. (1961), 'Visual memory test; The simulation of mental incompetence', *Archives of General Psychiatry, 4;* 79-83.

Beresford, S. (1995), *Motor Neurone Disease*, London: Chapman & Hall.

Berg I.J., Koning-Haanstra M & Deelman BG (1991) Long-term effects of memory rehabilitation: A controlled study. *Neuropsychological Rehabilitation, 1,* 91-111.

Berglund, M. & Risberg, J. (1980), 'Reversibility in alcohol dementia', in Begleiter, H. (ed.), *Biological Effects of Alcohol*, New York: Plenum.

Bernouilli, C., Seigfried, J., Baumgartner, G., Regli, F., et al. (1977), 'Danger of accidental person-to-person transmission of Creutzfeldt-Jakob disease by surgery', *The Lancet*, 1:131 478–9.

Biber, C., Butters, N. & Rosen, J. (1981), 'Encoding strategies and recognition of faces by alcoholic Korsakoff and other brain-damaged patients', *Journal of Clinical Neuropsychology*, 3: 315–30.

Binswanger, O. (1894), 'Die Abgrenzung der allgemeinen progressiven Paralyse' ('Distinguishing general progressive paralysis'), *Berliner klinische Wochenshrift*, 31: 1,137–9.

Blackburn, I. & Davidson, K. (1990), *Cognitive Therapy for Depression and Anxiety: A Practitioner's Guide* (1st reprint), Oxford: Blackwell.

Blessed, G., Tomlinson, B.E. & Roth, M. (1968), 'The association between a quantitative measure of dementia and of senile change in the cerebral grey matter of elderly subjects', *British Journal of Psychiatry*, 114: 797–811.

Bluglass, R. (1976), 'Malingering', in Krauss, S. (ed.), *Encyclopaedic Handbook of Medical Psychology*, London: Butterworths.

Bolt, J.M.W. (1970), 'Huntington's chorea in the West of Scotland', *British Journal of Psychiatry*, 116: 259–70.

Bolter, J.F. & Hannon, R. (1980), 'Cerebral damage associated with alcoholism: A reexamination', *The Psychological Record*, 30; 165–79.

Botwinick, J. (1977), 'Intellectual abilities', in Birren, J.E. & Schaie, K.W. (eds), *Handbook of the Psychology of Aging*, New York: Van Nostrand.

Botwinick, J. (1978), *Aging and Behavior*, (2nd edn), New York: Springer.

Botwinick, J. & Storandt, M. (1974), *Memory, Related Functions, and Age*, Springfield, Illinois: C.C. Thomas.

Botwinick, J. & Storandt, M. (1980), 'Recall and recognition of old information in relation to age and sex', *Journal of Gerontology, 35;* 70-76.

Bourgeois, M., Hébert, A. & Maisondieu, J. (1970), 'Depressive senile pseudo-dementia curable by electric shock', *Annales Médicopsychologique*, 128; 751–9.

Bouthet, C. (1995), 'Alzheimer's – focus', *Alzheimer's Research*, 1, 3: 107–8.

Bower, H.M. (1967), 'Sensory stimulation in the treatment of senile dementia', *Medical Journal of Australia*, 1: 1,113–19.

Braekus, A. (1995), 'A low, "normal" score on the Mini-Mental State Examination predicts development of dementia after three years', *Journal of The American Geriatrics Society*, 46: 656–61.

Braham, J. (1971), 'Jacob-Creutzfeldt disease: Treatment by amantadine', *British Medical Journal*, 4: 212–13.

Breg, W.R. (1977), 'A review of recent progress in research', *Pathobiology Annals*, 7: 257–303.

Breitner, J.C.S. & Folstein, M.F. (1984), 'Familial Alzheimer dementia: A prevalent disorder with specific clinical features', *Psychological Medicine*, 14: 63–80.

Briggs, A. (1972), *Report of the Committee on Nursing*, London: HMSO.

Brizzee, K.R., Ordy, J.M., Knox, C. & Jirge, S.K. (1980), 'Morphology and aging in the brain', in Maletta, G.J. & Pirozzolo, F.J. (Eds), *The Aging Nervous System*, New York: Praeger.

Brownell, B. & Oppenheimer, D.R. (1965), 'An ataxic form of subacute presenile polioencephalopathy (Creutzfeldt-Jakob disease)', *Journal of Neurology, Neurosurgery & Psychiatry*, 28: 350–61.

Bruhn, P., Arlien-Søborg, P., Gyldensted, C. & Christensen, E.L. (1981), 'Prognosis in chronic toxic encephalopathy', *Acta Neurologica Scandinavica*, 64: 259–72.

Brust, J.C.M. (1983), 'Vascular dementia – still overdiagnosed', *Stroke*, 14: 298–300.

Bucks R.S., Ashworth D.L., Wilcock G.K. & Siegfried K. (1996) Assessment of activities of daily living in dementia: Development of the Bristol Activities of Dailiy Living Scale. *Age & Ageing, 25*, 113-120.

Bucy, P.C. & Klüver, H. (1955), 'An anatomic investigation of the temporal lobe in monkey (*Macaca mulatta*)', *Journal of Complementary Neurology*, 103: 151–252.

Buelow, J.M. (1991), 'A correlation study of disabilities, stressors and coping methods in victims of multiple sclerosis', *Journal of Neuroscience Nursing*, 23, 4: 247–52.

Burger, P.C. & Vogel, F.S. (1973), 'The development of the pathologic changes of Alzheimer's disease and senile dementia in patients with Down's syndrome', *American Journal of Pathology*, 73:; 457–68.

Burish, T. & Bradley L.A. (1983), *Coping with Chronic Disease: Research and Applications*, London: Academic Press.

Burns, A.B. & Levy, R. (1994), *Dementia*, London: Chapman & Hall.

Burnside I (1990) Reminiscence: An independent nursing intervention. *Issues in Mental Health Nursing, 11* (1), 33-38.

Burnside, I. (1990), 'Reminiscence: An independent nursing

intervention', *Issues in Mental Health Nursing*, 11, 1: 33–8.

Butters, N. & Cermak, L.S. (1974), 'The role of cognitive factors in the memory disorders of alcoholic patients with the Korsakoff syndrome', *Annals of the New York Academy of Sciences*, 233: 61–75.

Butters, N. & Struss, A.T. (1989), 'Diencephalic amnesia', in Boller, F. & Grafman, J. (eds), *Handbook of Neuropsychology*, Vol. 3, Amsterdam: Elsevier.

Buzan, T. (1989), *Master Your Memory*, London: David Charles.

Cameron, D.E. (1967), 'Magnesium pemoline and human performance', *Science*, 157: 958–9.

Cameron, D.E. & Solyom, L. (1961), 'Effects of ribonucleic acid on memory', *Geriatrics*, 16: 74–81.

Caplan, L.R. & Schoene, W.C. (1978), 'Clinical features of subcortical arteriosclerotic encephalopathy (Binswanger disease)', *Neurology*, 28: 1,206–15.

Carlen, P.L., Wilkinson, D.A. & Wortzman, G. (1981), 'Cerebral atrophy and functional deficits in alcoholics without clinically apparent liver disease', *Neurology*, 31: 377–85.

Carney, M. (1983), 'Pseudodementia', *British Journal of Hospital Medicine*, 29: 312–18.

Charcot, J.M. (1877), *Lectures on the Diseases of the Nervous System Delivered at La Salpetriére*, London: New Sydenham Society.

Coates T.D. (1996) Dementia. *General Practitioner, 1 Mar*, 55-61.

Cohen NJ & Squire LR (1981) Preserved learning and retention of pattern analysing skill in amnesia: dissociation of knowing how and knowing that. *Science, 210*, 207-209.

Cole, G.M. & Timiras, P.S. (1987), 'Ubiquitin-protein conjugates in Alzheimer's lesions', *Neuroscience Letters*, 79: 207–12.

Collacott, R.A. (1992), 'The effect of age and residential placement on adaptive behaviour of adults with Down's syndrome', *British Journal of Psychiatry*, 161: 675–9.

Collacott, R.A. & Cooper, S. (1992), 'Adaptive behaviour after a depressive illness in Down's syndrome', *Journal of Nervous & Mental Disease*, 180: 468–70.

Collerton, D. (1986), 'Cholinergic function and intellectual decline in Alzheimer's disease', *Neuroscience*, 19: 1–28.

Collerton, D. (1993), 'Memory Disorders' in Greenwood, R., Barnes, M.P., McMillan, T.M. & Ward, C.D. (eds), *Neurological Rehabilitation*, Edinburgh: Churchill Livingstone.

Cook, R.H., Ward, B. & Austin, J. (1979), 'Studies in aging of the brain, Part IV – Familial Alzheimer's disease: Relation to transmissible dementia, aneuploidy and microtubular defects', *Neurology*, 29: 1,402–12.

Cooper, B. & Bickel, H. (1984), 'Population screening and the early detection of dementing disorders in old age: A review', *Psychological Medicine*, 14: 81–95.

Cooper, S. & Collacott, R.A. (1993), 'Prognosis of depression in Down's syndrome', *Journal of Nervous & Mental Disease*, 181: 204–5.

Cordell, B., Hoggins, L.S., Higaki, J., Zhong, Z., et al. (1995), 'A model of beta-amyloid formation and Alzheimer's disease', *Alzheimer's Research*, 1, 3: 111–16.

Corkin, S. (1982), 'Some relationships between global amnesias and the memory impairments in Alzheimer's disease', in Corkin, S., Davis, K.L., Growden, J.H., Usdin, E., et al. (eds), *Alzheimer's Disease: A Report of Research in Progress*, New York: Raven Press.

Corkin, S., Davis, K.L., Growdon, J.H., Usdin, E., et al. (1982), *'Alzheimer's Disease: A Report of Progress in Research – Aging'*, New York: Raven.

Corsellis, J.A.N., Bruton, C.J. & Freeman-Brown, D. (1973), 'The aftermath of boxing', *Psychological Medicine*, 3: 270–303.

Corsellis, J.A.N. & Evans, P.H. (1965), 'The relation of stenosis of the extracranial cerebral arteries to mental disorder and cerebral degeneration in old age', in Lühy, F. & Bischoff, A. (eds), *Proceedings of the Vth International Congress of Neuropathology*, Amsterdam: Excerpta Medica, 546–8.

Cosin, L.Z., Mort, M., Post, F., Westropp, C., et al. (1958), 'Experimental treatment of persistent senile confusion', *International Journal of Social Psychiatry*, 4: 24–42.

Cox, Y. (1993), 'Tailor-made job', *Nursing Times*, 89, 22: 66.

CPCS – Chichester Priority Care Services NHS Trust (1997) *Welcome to Chichester Priority Care Services*. SH1/25.04.97. Chichester, CPCS.

Craik, F.I.M. (1977), 'Age differences in human memory', in Birren, J.E. & Schaie, K.W. (eds), *Handbook of the Psychology of Aging*, New York: Van Nostrand.

Craik, F.I.M. (1994), 'Memory changes in normal aging', Current Directions in Psychological Science, 3; 5: 155-158.

Crapper, D.R., Dalton, A.L., Skopitz, M., Eng, P., et al. (1975), 'Alzheimer's degeneration in Down's syndrome', *Archives of Neurology*, 32: 618.

Creutzfeldt, H.G. (1920), 'Über eine eigenartige herdförmige Erkrankung des Zentralnervensystems' ('Concerning a strangely focused illness of the central nervous system'), *Zeitschrift für die gesamte Neurologie und Psychiatrie*, 57: 1–18.

Crook, T.H. & Larrabee, G.J. (1992), 'Normative data on a self-rating scale for evaluating memory in everyday life', *Archives of Clinical Neuropsychology*, 7: 45–51.

Crovitz, H., Harvey, M. & Horne, R. (1979), 'Problems in the acquisition of imagery mnemonics', *Cortex*, 15: 225–34.

Crystal, H., Dickson, D., Fuld, P. & Masur, D. (1988), 'Clinico-pathologic studies in dementia: Nondemented subjects with pathologically confirmed Alzheimer's disease', *Neurology*, 38, 11: 1,682–7.

Cullen, C. (1991), *Mental Handicap Nursing in the Context of 'Caring for People'*, London: Department of Health.

Cummings, J.L. (1986), 'Subcortical dementia: Neuropsychology, neuropsychiatry and pathophysiology', *British Journal of Psychiatry*, 149: 682–97.

Cummings, J.L. & Duchen, L.W. (1981), 'Klüver-Bucy syndrome in Pick's disease: Clinical and pathologic correlations', *Neurology* (New York), 31: 1,415–22.

Curran, S. & Wattis, J.P. (1989), 'Round-up: Searching for the cause of Alzheimer's disease', *Geriatric Medicine*, March: 13–14.

Cutler, N.R. (1985), 'Alzheimer's disease and Down's syndrome: New insights', *Annals of Internal Medicine*, 103: 556–78.

Daigneault, S. & Braun, C.M. (1993), 'Working memory and the self-ordered pointing task: further evidence of early prefrontal decline in normal aging', *Journal of Clinical and Experimental Neuropsychology, 15;* 6: 881-895.

Dale, G.E., Leigh, P.N., Luthert, P., Anderton, B.H. & Roberts, G.W. (1991), 'Neurofibrillary tangles in dementia pugilistica are ubiquitinated', *Journal of Neurology, Neurosurgery & Psychiatry*, 54: 116–18.

Dalton, A.J. (1992), *Alzheimer's Disease and Down's Syndrome*, Chichester: John Wiley.

Dalton, A.J., Crapper, D.R. & Schlotterer, G.R. (1974), 'Alzheimer's disease in Down's syndrome: Visual retention deficits', *Cortex*, 10: 366–77.

Damasio H & Damasio AR (1989) *Lesion Analysis in Neuropsychologia.* New York: Oxford University Press.

Damasio H & Damasio AR (1989) *Lesion Analysis in Neuropsychologia.* New York: Oxford University Press. Das, J.P. (1992), 'Beyond a multidimensional scale or merit', *Intelligence*, 16, 2: 137–49.

Das, J.P., Davison, M., Hiscox, M., Mishra, R.K., et al. (1993), 'Intellectual decline and aging: Individuals with Down's syndrome compared to other individuals with mental handicaps', *Report*, Edmonton: University of Alberta.

Das, J.P., Kirby, J.R. & Jarman, R. (1979), *Simultaneous and Successive Cognitive Processes*, New York: Academic Press.

Davies, S. (1996), 'Neuropsychological assessment of the older person', in Woods, R.T. (ed.), *Clinical Psychology of Ageing*, Chichester:

John Wiley.

Day, K.A. (1985), 'Psychiatric disorder in the middle aged and elderly mentally handicapped', *British Journal of Psychiatry*, December: 660–7.

Deary, I.J., Hunter R., Langan, S.J. & Goodwin, G.M. (1991), 'Inspection time, psychometric intelligence and clinical estimates of cognitive ability in presenile Alzheimer's disease and Korsakoff's psychosis', *Brain*, 114: 2,543–54.

Deary, I.J. & Whalley, L.J. (1988), 'Recent research on the causes of Alzheimer's disease', *British Medical Journal*, 297: 807–9.

Delabar, J.M., Goldgaber, D., Laqmour, Y., Nicole, A., et al. (1987), 'Beta amyloid gene duplication in Alzheimer's disease and karyotypically normal Down's syndrome', *Science*, 235: 1,390–2.

Denney, N.W. (1974), 'Evidence for developmental changes in categorization for children and adults', *Human Development*, 17: 41–53.

Dickson, D.W. (2001), 'Neuropathology of Alzheimer's disease and other dementias', *Clinics in Geriatric Medicine, 17;* 2: 209-228.

Down, J.L. (1866), 'Observations on an ethnic classification of idiots', *London Hospitals Reports*, London: London Hospitals.

Dudek, F.J. (1979), 'The continuing misinterpretation of the standard error of measurement', *Psychological Bulletin*, 86: 335–7.

Duffy, P., Wolf, J., Collins, G., De Voe, A.G. et al. (1974), 'Possible person-to-person transmission of Creutzfeldt-Jakob disease', *New England Journal of Medicine*, 290: 692–3.

Dunn, L.M. & Dunn, L.M. (1981), *Peabody Picture Vocabulary Test – Revised*, Minnesota: American Guidance Service.

Eagger, S.A., Levy, R. & Sahakian, B.J. (1991), 'Tacrine in Alzheimer's disease', *The Lancet*, 337: 989–92.

Earles, J.L. & Salthouse, T.A. (1995), 'Interrelations of age, health, and speed', *Journal of Gerontology, 50;* 1: P33-P41.

Earll, L., Johnston, M. & Mitchell, E. (1993), 'Coping with motor neurone disease – an analysis using self-regulation theory', *Palliative Medicine*, 7, Supplement 2: 20–1.

Edwards, A.E. & Hart, G.M. (1974), 'Hyperbaric oxygenation and the cognitive functioning of the aged', *Journal of the American Geriatrics Society*, 22: 376–9.

Eich, E. (1984), 'Memory for unattended events: Remembering with and without awareness', *Memory & Cognition*, 12: 105–11.

Ellis, R.D., Goldberg, J.H. & Detweiler, M.C. (1996), 'Predicting age-related differences in visual information processing using two-stage queing model', *Journal of Gerontology, 51;* 3: P155-P65.

Ellis, N.C. & Hennelley, R.A. (1980), 'A bilingual word-length effect: Implications for intelligence testing and the relative ease of mental calculation in Welsh and English', *British Journal of Psychology*, 71: 43–52.

Ellis, W.G., McCulloch, J.R. & Corley, C.L. (1974), 'Presenile dementia in Down's syndrome: Ultrastructural identity with Alzheimer's disease', *Neurology (Minneapolis)*, 24: 101–6.

Enoch, M.D., Trethowan, W.H. & Barker, J.C. (1967), *Some Uncommon Psychiatric Syndromes*, Bristol: John Wright.

Erickson, R.C. (1978), 'Problems in the clinical assessment of memory', *Experimental Aging Research*, 4: 255–72.

Esiri, M. (1991), 'Neuropathology', in Jacoby, R. & Oppenheimer, C. (eds), *Psychiatry in the Elderly*, Oxford: Oxford Medical Publications.

Esterling, B., Kiecolt-Glaser, J.K., Bodnar, J. & Glaser, R. (1994), 'Chronic stress, social support, and persistent alterations in the nature killer cell response to cytokines in older adults', *Health Psychology*, 13: 291–9.

Evans, M. (1975), 'Cerebral disorders due to drugs of dependence and hallucinogens,' in Rankin, J.G. (ed.), *Alcohol, Drugs and Brain Damage*, Toronto: Addiction Research Foundation.

Evenhuis, H.M. (1992), 'Evaluation of a screening instrument for dementia in ageing mentally retarded persons', *Journal of Intellectual Disability Research*, 36: 37–47.

Evenhuis, H.M. (1992a), *'Provisional Manual of the Dementia Questionnaire for Mentally Retarded Persons (DMR)'*, Zwammerdam: Hooge Burch.

Evenhuis, H.M. (1992b), 'Evaluation of a screening instrument for dementia in ageing mentally retarded persons', *Journal of Intellectual Disability Research, 36:* 337-347.

Evenhuis, H.M., Kengen, M.M.F. & Eurlings, H.A.L. (1990), *Dementie Vragenlijst Zwakzinnigen* (Dementia Questionnaire for the Mentally Deficient), Zwammerdam: Hooge Burch.

Eyman, R.K., Call, T.L. & White, J.F. (1991), 'Life expectancy of persons with Down's syndrome', *American Journal of Mental Retardation*, 95: 603–12.

Eyman, R.K., Grossman, H.J., Tarjan, G. & Miller, C.R. (1987), 'Life expectancy and mental retardation: A longitudinal study in a state residential facility', *Monographs of the American Association on Mental Deficiency*, 7: 1–73.

Farrell, M.J. & Kaufman, M.R. (1943), 'A compendium on neuropsychiatry in the army', *Army Medical Bulletin*, 66: 1–112.

Feinberg, T. & Goodman, B. (1984), 'Affective illness, dementia and pseudo-dementia', *Journal of Clinical Psychiatry*, 45: 99–103.

Feldman, R.G., Chandler, K., Levy, L. & Glaser, G. (1963), 'Familial Alzheimer's disease', *Neurology*, 13: 811–20.

Feldman, H., Sauter, A., Donald, A., Gélinas, I., Gauthier, S., Torfs, K., Parys, W. & Mehnert, A. (2001) The Disability Assessment for Dementia Scale: A 12-month study of functional ability in mild to moderate severity Alzheimer disease. *Alzheimer Disease & Associated Disorders, 15* (2), 89-95.

Fischman, H.K., Reisberg, B., Albu, P., Ferris, S.H., et al. (1984), 'Sister chromatid exchanges and cell cycle kinetics in Alzheimer's disease', *Biological Psychiatry*, 19, 3: 319–27.

Fisk, A.D., Rogers, W.A., Cooper, B.P. & Gilbert, D.K. (1997), 'Automatic category search and its transfer: aging, type of search, and level of learning', *Journal of Gerontology, 52;* 2: P91-P102.

Fisman, M. (1985), 'Pseudodementia', *Progress in Neuro-Psychopharmacology & Biological Psychiatry*, 9: 481–4.

Folstein, M., Anthony, J.C. & Parhad, I. (1985), 'The meaning of cognitive impairment in the elderly', *Journal of the American Geriatric Society*, 33: 228–35.

Folstein, M., Folstein, S. & McHugh, P.R. (1975), 'Mini-mental state: a practical method for grading the cognitive state of patients for the clinician', *Journal of Psychiatric Research*, 12: 189–98.

Fraser, M. (1988), *Dementia: Its Nature and Management*, Chichester: John Wiley: 5–20. Fraser, J. & Mitchell, A. (1876), 'Kalmuc idiocy: Report of a case with autopsy with notes on 62 cases', *Journal of Mental Science*, 22: 161.

Fromholt, P. & Larsen, S.F. (1991), 'Autobiographical memory in normal aging and primary degenerative dementia (dementia of Alzheimer type)', *Journal of Gerontology (Psychological Sciences)*, 46, 3: 85–91.

Fryers, T. (1986), 'Survival in Down's syndrome', *Journal of Mental Deficiency Research*, 30: 101–10.

Furster, J.M. (1993), 'Frontal lobes', Current Opinions in Neurobiology, 3; 160-165.

Gale, J. & Livesley, B. (1974), 'Attitudes towards geriatrics: A report of the King's survey', *Age & Aging*, 3: 49–53.

Ganser, S.J.M. (1898), 'Ueber einen eigenartigen hysterischen Daemmerzustand' ('Concerning a strangely hysterical state of dopiness'), *Archiv für Psychiatrie und Nervenkrankheiten*, 30: 633–40.

Garcia, C.A., Reding, M.J. & Blass, J.P. (1981), 'Overdiagnosis of dementia', *Journal of the American Geriatrics Society*, 29: 407–10.

Gardiner, J.M., Gawlik, B. & Richardson-Klavehn, A. (1994), 'Maintenance rehearsal affects knowing, not remembering: Elaborative rehearsal affects remembering, not knowing', *Psychonomic Bulletin*, 1, 1: 107–10.

Gardner H (1977) *The Shattered Mind: The Person after Brain Damage*. London: Routledge & Kegan Paul.

Gath, A. (1986), 'Ageing and mental handicap', *Developmental and Child Neurology*, 28: 515–24.

Gatz, M. & Pearson, C.G. (1988), 'Ageism revised and the provision of psychological services', *American Psychologist*, 43: 184–8.

Gélinas, I., Gauthier, L., McIntyre, M. & Gauthier, S. (1999) Development of a functional measure for persons with Alzheimer's disease: The Disability Asessment for Dementia. *American Journal of Occupational Therapy, 53* (5), 471-481.

Gibbs, C.J., Gajdusek, D.C., Asher, D.M., Alpers, M.P. et al. (1968), 'Creutzfeldt-Jakob disease (spongiform encephalopathy): Transmission to the chimpanzee', *Science*, 161: 388–9.

Gibson, H.B. (1991), *The Emotional and Sexual Lives of Older People*, London: Chapman & Hall.

Giles GM & Clark-Wilson J (1993) *Brain Injury Rehabilitation: A Neurofunctional Approach*. London: Chapman & Hall.

Gilleard, C.J. (1984) *Problem checklist and strain scale*. London: Croom Helm.

Glasgow, R.E., Zeiss, R.A., Barrera, M. & Lewinsohn, P.M. (1977), 'Case studies on remediating memory deficits', *Journal of Clinical Psychology*, 33: 1,049–54.

Glisky, E.L., Schacter, D.L. & Tulving, E. (1986), 'Computer learning by memory impaired patients: Acquisition and retention of complex knowledge', *Neuropsychologia*, 24: 313–28.

Glisky, E.L. & Schacter, D.L. (1988), 'Long term retention of computer learning by patients with memory disorders', *Neuropsychologia*, 26: 173–8.

Glisky EL, Schacter DL & Tulving E (1986) Computer learning by memory impaired patients: Acquisition and retention of complex knowledge. *Neuropsychologia, 24,* 313-328.

Godfrey, H.P. & Knight, R.G. (1987), 'Intervention for amnesics: A review', *British Journal of Clinical Psychology*, 26, 2: 83–91.

Goldberg, D.P. & Williams P. (1988). *General Health Questionnaire, GHQ12*. Windsor, NFER-NELSON.

Golding, E. (1989), *The Middlesex Elderly Assessment of Mental State*, Bury St Edmunds: Thames Valley Test Co.

Goodall, A., Drage, T. & Bell, G. (1995), *The Bereavement and Loss Training Manual*, Bicester: Winslow Press.

Gordon, W.A. (1987), 'Methodological consideration in cognitive remediation', in Meier, M.J., Benton, A.L. & Diller, L. (eds), *Neuropsychological Remediation*, Edinburgh: Churchill Livingstone.

Goudie, F. (1993), 'Problems of aging', in Stokes, G. & Goudie, F. (eds), *Working with Dementia*, Oxford: Winslow Press.

Granger, C.V. & Greer, D.S. (1976), 'Functional status measurement and medical rehabilitation outcomes', *Archives of Physical Medicine Rehabilitation*, 58: 103–9.

Green, J.B. (1991), *Dealing with Death: Practices and Procedures*, London: Chapman & Hall.

Gregersen, P., Middelsen, S. & Klausen, H. (1978), ('A chronic cerebral syndrome in painters: Dementia due to inhalation or cryptogenic origin?'), *Ugeskrift for Läeger*, 140: 1,638–44.

Gulick, E.E. (1994), 'Social support among persons with multiple sclerosis', *Research in Nursing and Health*, 17: 195–206.

Guterman, A. & Smith, R.W. (1987), 'Neurological sequelae of boxing', *Sports Medicine*, 4: 194–210.

Haberland, C. (1969), 'Alzheimer's disease in Down's syndrome: Clinical-neuropathological observations', *Acta Neurologica*, 69: 369–80.

Hachinski, V.C. (1983), 'Differential diagnosis of Alzheimer's dementia: Multi-infarct dementia', in Reisberg, B. (ed.), *Alzheimer's Disease*, New York: The Free Press, 188–92.

Hachinski, V.C., Iliff, L., Zilhka, E., DuBoulay, G.H., et al. (1975), 'Cerebral blood flow in dementia', *Archives of Neurology*, 32: 632–7.

Hagberg, B. & Gustafson, L. (1985), 'On diagnosis of dementia: Psychometric investigation and clinical psychiatric evaluation in relation to verified diagnosis', *Archives of Gerontology & Geriatrics*, 4: 321–32.

Haggar, L. & Hutchinson, R. (1991), 'Snoezelen: An approach to the provision of a leisure resource for people with profound and multiple handicaps', *Mental Handicap*, 19: 51–5.

Hampshire Social Services (1989), *Hampshire Social Services Assessment*, Southampton: Hampshire Social Services.

Hanley, I. & Baikie, E. (1984), 'Understanding and treating depression in the elderly', in Hanley, I. & Hodge, J. (eds), *Psychological Approaches to the Care of the Elderly*, Beckenham: Croom Helm.

Hanley, I.G. & Lusty, K. (1984), 'Case histories and shorter communications: Aids in reality orientation', *Behaviour Research & Therapy*, 22, 6: 709–12.

Hansch, E.C., Syndulko, K. & Pirozzolo, F.J. (1980), 'Electrophysiological measurement in aging and in death', in Maletta, G.J. & Pirozzolo, F.J. (eds), *The Aging Nervous System*, New York: Praeger.

Harrison, M.J. (1983), *Contemporary Neurology*, London: Butterworths.

Hart, S. (1988), 'Language and dementia: A review', *Psychological Medicine*, 18: 99–112.

Hartley, X.Y. (1982), 'Receptive language processing in Down's syndrome children', *Journal of Mental Deficiency Research*, 26: 263–9.

Haste H & Gregory R (1993) Quizzical answers. *The Psychologist, Apr,* 191-192.

Haxby, J.V. (1985), 'Clinical and neuropsychological studies of dementia in Down's syndrome', *Annals of Internal Medicine*, 103: 572–4.

Haxby, J.V. (1989), 'Neuropsychological evaluation of adults with Down's syndrome: Patterns of selective impairment in non-demented old adults', *Journal of Mental Deficiency Research*, 33: 193–210.

Haycox, J. (1984), 'A simple reliable clinical behavioral scale for assessing demented patients', *Journal of Clinical Psychiatry*, 45: 23–4.

Heard, R.N.S. (1993), 'New horizons in the treatment of multiple sclerosis', *The Medical Journal of Australia*, May, 158, 17: 714–16.

Heathfield, K.W.G. (1967), 'Huntington's chorea', *Brain*, 90: 203–32.

Henderson, A.S. & Huppert, F.A. (1985), 'The problem of mild dementia', *Psychological Medicine*, 14: 5–11.

Heston, L.L. (1977), 'Alzheimer's disease, trisomy 21, and myeloproliferative disorders: Associations suggesting a genetic diathesis', *Science, 196:* 322-323.

Heston, L.L., Mastri, A.R., Anderson, V.E. & White, J. (1981), 'Dementia of the Alzheimer type: Clinical genetics, natural history and associated conditions', *Archives of General Psychiatry*, 38: 1,085–90.

Hewitt, K.E., Carter, G. & Jancar, J. (1985), 'Ageing in Down's syndrome', *British Journal of Psychiatry*, 147: 58–62.

Heyman, A., Wilkinson, W.E., Stafford, J.A., Helms, M.J., et al. (1984), 'Alzheimer's disease: A study of epidemiological aspects', *Annals of Neurology*, 15: 335–41.

Hicks, L.H. & Birren, J.E. (1970), 'Aging, brain damage, and psychomotor slowing', *Psychological Bulletin*, 74: 377–96.

Hodges JR & McCarthy RA (1993) Autobiographical amnesia resulting from bilateral paramedial thalamic function. *Brain, 116,* 921-940.

Hogg, J., Moss, S. & Cooke, D. (1988a), *Ageing and Mental Handicap*, London: Chapman & Hall.

Hogg, J., Moss, S. & Cooke, D. (1988b), 'From mid-life to old age: Ageing and the nature of specific life-transitions of people with mental handicap', in Horobin, G. & May, D. (Eds), *Living with Mental Handicap: Transitions in the Lives of People with Mental Handicap*, London: Jessica Kingsley.

Holden, U. (1989), *Neuropsychology and Ageing*, London: Chapman & Hall.

Howieson, D.B. (1980), 'Confabulation', paper presented at North

Pacific Society of Neurology & Psychiatry, Bend, Oregon, March.

HSS - Hampshire Social Services (1989), *'Hampshire Social Services Assessment'*, Southampton: Hampshire Social Services.

Huber, S.J., Paulson, G.W. & Shuttleworth, E.C. (1987), 'Magnetic imaging correlates of dementia in multiple sclerosis', *Archives of Neurology*, 44: 732–6.

Hughes, C.P., Berg, L. & Danziger, W.L. (1982), 'A new clinical scale for the staging of dementia', *British Journal of Psychiatry*, 140: 566–72.

Hulme, C., Lee, G. & Brown, G.D.A. (1993), 'Short-term memory impairments in Alzheimer-type dementia: Evidence for separable impairments of articulatory rehearsal and long-term memory', *Neuropsychologia*, 31: 161–72.

Hulsegge, J. & Verheul, A. (1987), *Snoezelen*, Chesterfield: ROMPA.

Humphreys, G.W. & Bruce, V. (1989), *Visual Cognition: Computational, Experimental and Neuropsychological Perspectives*, New Jersey: Lawrence Erlbaum.

Huntington, G. (1872), 'On chorea', *Medical & Surgical Reporter* (Philadelphia), 26: 317–21.

Huppert, F.A. & Tym, E. (1986), 'Clinical and neuropsychological assessment of dementia', *British Medical Bulletin*, 42, 1: 11–18.

Hussain, R.A. (1981), *Geriatric Psychology: A Behavioural Perspective*, London: Van Nostrand.

Hutchinson, R. (1991), *The Whittington Hall Snoezelen Project: A Report from Inception to the First Twelve Months*, Chesterfield: North Derbyshire Health Authority.

Ineichen, B. (1989), *Senile Dementia*, London: Chapman & Hall.

Inglis, J. (1959), 'Learning, retention and conceptual usage in elderly patients with memory disorder', *Journal of Abnormal Social Psychology*, 59: 210–15.

Itzin, C. (1986), 'Ageism awareness training: A model for group work', in Phillipson, C., Bernard, M. & Strang, P. (eds), *Dependency and Interdependency in Old Age: Theoretical Perspectives and Policy Alternatives*, Beckenham: Croom Helm.

Jacobs, L., Winter, P.M., Alvis, H.J. & Small, S.M. (1969), 'Hyperoxygenation effect on cognitive functioning in the aged', *New England Journal of Medicine*, 281: 753–7.

Jakob, A. (1921), 'Über eine eigenartige Erkrankungen des Zentralnervensystems mit bemerkenswertem anatomischen Befunde' ('Concerning a strange illness of the central nervous system with noteworthy anatomical findings'), *Zeitschrift für die gesamte Neurologie und Psychiatrie*, 64: 147–228.

Jalowiec, A. & Powers, M.J. (1981), 'Stress and coping in hypertensive and emergency room patients', *Nursing Research*, 30, 1: 10–15.

Jancar, J. (1984), 'Protracted survival in patients with Down's syndrome', *British Medical Journal*, 288: 152. Jay, P. (1979), *Report of the Committee of Enquiry into Mental Handicap Nursing and Care*, London: HMSO.

Jernigan, T., Zatz, I.M. & Feinberg, K. (1980), 'Measurement of Cerebral Atrophy in the Aged' in Poon, L.W. (ed), *Aging in the 1980s. Psychological Issues*, Washington D.C.: American Psychological Corporation.

Jervis, G.A. (1948), 'Early senile dementia in mongoloid idiocy', *American Journal of Psychiatry, 105:* 102-106.

Jones, D.P. & Nevin, S. (1954), 'Rapidly progressive cerebral degeneration (subacute vascular encephalopathy) with mental disorder, focal disturbances and myoclonic epilepsy', *Journal of Neurology, Neurosurgery & Psychiatry*, 17: 148–59.

Jones, R. (1987), 'Applicability of the WAIS-R: Its use with people with mental handicap', *Mental Handicap*, 15, 4: 155–8.

Jorm, A.F. (1987), *Understanding Senile Dementia*, London: Chapman & Hall.

Jorm, A.F. (1990), *'The Epidemiology of Alzheimer's Disease and Related Disorders'*, London: Chapman & Hall.

Jorm, A.F. (1990), *The Epidemiology of Alzheimer's Disease and Related Disorders*, London: Chapman & Hall. Kahana, E., Alter, M., Braham, J. & Sofer, D. (1974), 'Creutzfeldt-Jakob disease: Focus among Libyan Jews in Israel', *Science*, 183: 90–1.

Kang, J., Lemaire, H.G., Unterbeck, A., Selbaum, J.M., *et al.*. (1987), 'The precursor of Alzheimer's disease amyloid A4 protein resembles a cell surface receptor', *Nature, 235:* 733-736.

Kapur N (1991) Amnesia in relation to fugue states - distinguishing a neurological from a psychogenic basis. *British Journal of Psychiatry, 159,* 872-877.

Kapur N (1993) Transient epileptic amnesia - a clinical update and a reformulation. *Journal of Neurology, Neurosurgery & Psychiatry, 56,* 1184-1190.

Kapur, N. (1994), *Memory Disorders in Clinical Practice*, Hove: Lawrence Erlbaum.

Kapur N, Ellison D, Smith MP, McLellan DL & Burrows EH (1992) Focal retrograde amnesia following bilateral temporal lobe pathology: A neuropsychological and magnetic resonance study. *Brain, 115,* 73-85.

Kapur N, Scholey K, Moore E, Baker S, Brice J, Thompson SBN, Shiel A, Carn P, Abbott P & Fleming J (1996a) Long-term retention deficits in two cases of disproportionate retrograde amnesia. *Journal of Cognitive Neuroscience, 8* (5), 416-434.

Kapur, N., Thompson, S.B.N., Cook, P., Lang, D. & Brice, J. (1996),

'Anterograde but not retrograde memory loss following combined mammilliary body and medial thalamic lesions', *Neuropsychologia, 34;* 1: 1-8.

Karlsson, T., Backman, L., Herlitz, A. & Neilsson, L.G. (1989), 'Memory involvement at different stages', *Neuropsychologia*, 27, 5: 737–42.

Kaszniak, A.W. (1986), 'The neuropsychology of dementia', in *Neuropsychological Assessment of Neuropsychiatric Disorders*, New York: Oxford University Press.

Kato, T., Katagiri, T., Hirano, T., Kawanami, T., et al. (1989), 'Lewy body-like inclusions in sporadic motor neuron disease are ubiquitinated', *Acta Neuropathologica* (Berlin), 77: 391–6.

Katona, C. (1989), *Dementia Disorders*, London: Chapman & Hall.

Katzman, R. (1976), 'The prevalence and malignancy of Alzheimer's disease', *Archives of Neurology*, 33; 217–18.

Katzman, R. & Karasu, T.B. (1975), 'Differential diagnosis of dementia', in Fields, W.S. (ed.), *Neurological and Sensory Disorders in the Elderly*, Miami: Symposia Specialists.

Kay, B. (1993), 'Keeping it in the family', *Nursing Times*, 89, 22: 64–5.

Kendrick, D. (1985), *Kendrick Cognitive Tests for the Elderly: Manual*, Windsor: NFER-Nelson.

Kennedy, A. (1959), 'Psychological factors in confusional states in the elderly', *Geriontologia Clinica*, 1: 71–82.

Kennedy, A. & Neville, J. (1957), 'Sudden loss of memory', *British Medical Journal*, 2: 428–33.

Kiecolt-Glaser, J.K., Dura, J.R., Speicher, C.E., Trask, O.J., et al. (1991), 'Spousal caregivers of dementia victims: Longitudinal changes in immunity and health', *Psychosomatic Medicine*, 53: 345–62.

Kiecolt-Glaser, J.K., Marucha, P.K., Malarkey, W.B., Marcado, A.M., et al. (1995), 'Slowing of wound healing by psychological stress', *The Lancet*, 346: 1,194–6.

Kiloh, L.G. (1961), 'Pseudo-dementia', *Acta Psychiatrica Scandinavica*, 37: 75–81.

Klüver, H. & Bucy, P.C. (1930), 'Preliminary analysis of functions of the temporal lobes in monkeys', *Archives of Neurology & Psychiatry*, 42: 979–1,000.

Knight, R.G., Godfrey, H.P.D. & Shelton, E.J. (1988), 'The psychological deficits associated with Parkinson's disease', *Clinical Psychology Review*, 8: 391–410.

Kolata, G. (1985), 'Down's syndrome – Alzheimer's linked', *Science*, 230: 1,152–3.

Kopelman, M.D. (1985), 'Rates of forgetting in Alzheimer-type dementia and Korsakoff's syndrome', *Neuropsychologia*, 23: 623–8.

Kopelman, M.D. (1989), 'Remote and autobiographical memory, temporal context memory and frontal atrophy in Korsakoff and Alzheimer patients', *Neuropsychologia*, 27: 437–60.

Kopelman, M.D. (1994), 'Working memory in the amnesic syndrome and degenerative dementia', *Neuropsychology*, 8, 4: 555–62.

Kopelman, M.D., Wilson, B.A. & Baddeley, A.D. (1990), *The Autobiographical Memory Interview*, Bury St Edmunds: Thames Valley Test Co.

Kovach, C.R. (1990), 'Promise and problems in reminiscence research', *Journal of Gerontology*, 16, 4: 10–14.

Kovanen, J., Haltia, M. & Cantell, K. (1980), 'Failure of interferon to modify Creutzfeldt-Jakob disease', *British Medical Journal*, 280: 902.

Kramer, N.A. & Jarvik, L. (1979), 'Assessment of intellectual changes in the elderly', in Raskin, A. & Jarvik, L. (eds), *Psychiatric Symptoms and Cognitive Loss in the Elderly*, Washington, DC: Hemisphere.

Kräupl-Taylor, F. (1966), *Psychopathology: Its Causes and Symptoms*, London: Butterworths.

Kroll, P., Seigl, R., O'Neill, B. & Edwards, R.P. (1980), 'Cerebral cortical atrophy in alcoholic men', *Journal of Clinical Psychiatry*, 41: 417–21.

Kumar, A. & Gottlieb, G.L. (1993), 'Frontotemporal dementias: A new clinical syndrome?', *American Journal of Geriatric Psychiatry*, 1, 2: 95–107.

Kuriansky, J.B. (1976), 'The assessment of self-care capacity in geriatric patients by objective and subjective methods', *Journal of Clinical Psychology*, 32: 95–102.

Kurleycheck, R.T. (1983), 'Use of a digital alarm chronograph as a memory aid', *Clinical Gerontologist*, 1: 93–4.

Kuusisto, J., Kiovisto, K. & Kervinen, K. (1994), 'Association of apolipoprotein E phenotypes with the late onset Alzheimer's disease: Population based study', *British Medical Journal*, 309: 636–8.

Kuzuhara, S., Mori, H., Izumiyama, N., Yoshimura, M., et al. (1988), 'Lewy bodies are ubiquitinated', *Acta Neuropathologica (Berlin)*, 75: 345–53.

Lai, F. & Williams, R.S. (1989), 'A prospective study of Alzheimer disease in Down syndrome', *Archives of Neurology*, 46: 849–53.

Lambert, G.J. & Bieliauskas, L.A. (1993), 'Distinguishing between depression and dementia in the elderly: A review of neuropsychological findings', *Archives of Clinical Neuropsychology*, 8: 149–70.

Lamberty, G.J. & Bieliauskas, L.A. (1993), 'Distinguishing between depression and dementia in the elderly: A review of neuropsychological findings', *Archives of Clinical Neuropsychology*,

8: 149-170.

La Rue, M. (1982), 'Memory loss and ageing', *Psychiatric Clinics of North America*, 5: 89–103.

Larsson, T., Sjögren, T. & Jacobson, G. (1963), 'Senile dementia: A clinical, sociomedical and genetic study', *Acta Psychiatrica Scandinavica*, 39, Supplement: 167.

Lassen, P.D. (1990), 'Psychosocial adjustment in multiple sclerosis', *Rehabilitation Nursing*, 15, 5: 242–6.

Lauter, H. & Meyer, J.E. (1968), 'Clinical and nosological concepts of senile dementia', in Miller, C. & Ciompi, L. (Eds), *Senile Dementia: Clinical and Therapeutic Aspects*, Berne: Hans Huber.

Lawton, M.P. & Brody, E.C. (1969), 'Assessment of old people: self-maintain-ing and instrumental activities of daily living', *Gerontologist*, 9: 179–86.

Leber, P. (1986), 'Establishing the efficacy of drugs with psychogeriatric indications', in Cook, T., Bartus, R., Ferris, S. and Gershon, S. (eds), *Geriatric Psychopharmacology*, New Canaan: Mark Powley Associates.

Leckliter, I.N., Matarazzo, J.D. & Silverstein, A.B. (1986), 'A literature review of factor analytic studies of the WAIS-R', *Journal of Clinical Psychology*, 42: 332–42.

Lee, K.H., Hashimoto, S.A., Hooge, J.P., Kastrukoft, L.F., et al. (1991), 'Magnetic resonance imaging of the head in the diagnosis of multiple sclerosis: A prospective 2 year follow-up and comparison of clinical evaluation, evoked potentials, oligoclonal banding and CT', *Neurology*, 41: 657–60.

Leigh, P.N., Anderton, G.H., Dodson, A., Gallo, J., et al. (1988), 'Ubiquitin deposits in anterior horn cells in motor neurone disease', *Neuroscience Letters*, 93: 197–203.

Leigh, P.N., Pobst, A., Dale, G.E., Power, D.P., et al. (1989), 'New aspects of the pathology of neurodegenerative disorders as revealed by ubiquitin antibodies', *Acta Neuropathologica (Berlin)*, 79: 61–72.

Lennox, G., Lowe, J., Morrell, K., Langdon, M., et al. (1988), 'Ubiquitin is a component of neurofibrillary tangles in a variety of neurodegenerative diseases', *Neuroscience Letters*, 94: 211–17.

Leuchter, A.F., Newton, T.F., Cook, I.A., Walter, D.O., et al. (1992), 'Changes in brain functional connectivity in Alzheimer-type and multi-infarct dementia', *Brain*, 115: 1,543–61.

Leventhal, H., Nerenz, D. & Steele, D.J. (1984), 'Illness representations and coping with health threats', in Baum, A., Taylor, S.E. & Singer, J.E. (eds), *Handbook of Psychology and Health, Vol. IV: Social Psychological Aspects of Health*, New Jersey: Lawrence Erlbaum.

Levinson, A., Friedman, A. & Stamps, F. (1955), 'Variability of mongolism', *Paediatrics*, 16: 43–54.

Levinson, A., Friedman, A. & Stamps, F. (1955), 'Variability of mongolism', *Paediatrics, 16:* 43-54.

Lezak, M.D. (1983), *'Neuropsychological Assessment, 2nd ed'*, New York: Oxford University Press.

Lezak MD (1995) *Neuropsychological Assessment. 3rd Edn.* Oxford: Oxford University Press.

Light, E., Niederhe, G. & Lebowitz, B.D. (Eds) (1994), *Stress Effects on Family Caregivers of Alzheimer's Patients*, New York: Springer.

Linn, M.W. & Linn, B.S. (1983), 'Assessing activities of daily living in institutional settings', in Cook, T., Ferris, R. & Bartus, R. (eds), *Assessment in Geriatric Psychopharmacology*, New Canaan: Mark Powley Associates.

Lishman, W.A. (1981), 'Cerebral disorder in alcoholism syndromes of impairment', *Brain*, 104: 1–20.

Lishman, W.A. (1983), *Organic Psychiatry: The Psychological Consequences of Cerebral Disorder*, Oxford: Blackwell.

Lishman, W.A. (1987), *Organic Psychiatry: The Psychological Consequences of Cerebral Disorder* (2nd edn), Oxford: Blackwell.

Long, A.P. & Haig, L. (1992), 'How do clients benefit from Snoezelen? An exploratory study', *British Journal of Occupational Therapy*, 55, 3: 103–6.

Lord, F.M. & Novick, M.R. (1968), *Statistical Theories of Mental Test Scores*, Massachusetts: Addison-Wesley.

Lorge, I. (1936), 'The influence of the test upon the nature of mental decline as a function of age', *Journal of Educational Psychology*, 27: 100–10.

Lowe, J., Blanchard, A. & Morrell, K. (1988), 'Ubquitin is a common factor in intermediate filament inclusion bodies of diverse type in man, including those of Parkinson's disease, Pick's disease, and Alzheimer's disease, as well as Rosenthal Fibres in cerebellar astrocytomas, cytoplasmic bodies in muscle, and mallory bodies in alcoholic liver disease', *Journal of Pathology*, 155: 9–15.

Lowe, J., Lennox, G. & Jefferson, D. (1988), 'A filamentous inclusion body within anterior horn neurones in motor neurone disease defined by immunocytochemical localisation of ubiquitin', *Neuroscience Letters*, 94: 203–10.

Lucotte, G., Turpin, J. & Raisonnier, A. (1995), 'Association of apolipoprotein E4 allele with late and early Alzheimer's disease, but not with vascular dementia or Parkinson's disease, in French patients', *Alzheimer's Research*, 1, 3: 145–6.

Luria, A.R. (1966), *Human Brain and Psychological Processes*, New York: Harper & Row.

Luscombe G., Brodaty, H. & Freeth, S. (1998) Younger people with dementia: Diagnostic issues, effects on carers and use of services. *International Journal of Geriatric Psychiatry, 13* (5), 323-330.

Lusins, J., Zimberg, S., Smokler, H. & Gurley, K. (1980), 'Alcoholism and cerebral atrophy: A study of 50 patients with CT scan and psychologic testing', *Alcoholism*, 4: 406–11.

Lyon, R.L. (1962), 'Huntington's chorea in the Moray Firth area', *British Medical Journal*, 1: 1,301–6.

MacInnes, W. (1983), 'Ageing and dementia', in Golden, C.J., Moses, J.A. Jr, Coffman, J.C., Miller, W.R. & Strider, F.D. (Eds), *Clinical Neuropsychology*, New York: Grune & Stratton.

Maclean, W.E., Ellis, D.N., Galbreath, H.N., Halpern, L.F., *et al..* (1991), 'Rhythmic motor behaviour of preambulatory motor impaired, Down syndrome and nondisabled children - A comparative analysis', *Journal of Abnormal Child Psychology, 19:* 319-330.

Macmillan, D. (1960), 'Preventive geriatrics: Opportunity of a community mental health service', *The Lancet*, 2: 1,439–41.

Mahendra, B. (1985), 'Depression and dementia: The multi-faceted relationship', *Psychological Medicine*, 15: 227–36.

Mahler, M.E. (1992), 'Behavioral manifestations associated with multiple sclerosis', *Psychiatric Clinics of North America*, 15, 2: 427–38.

Mahoney, F.I. & Barthel, D.W. (1965), 'Functional evaluation: The Barthel index', *Maryland State Medical Journal*, 14: 61–5.

Malamud, N. (1972), 'Neuropathology of organic brain syndrome: Syndromes associated with aging', in Gaitz, C.M. (ed.), *Aging and the Brain* (3rd edn), New York: Plenum.

Mann, D.M.A. (1995), 'How genetic causes of Alzheimer's disease further our understanding of its pathogenesis', *Alzheimer's Research*, 1, 3: 117–22.

Martland, H.S. (1928), 'Punch drunk', *Journal of the American Medical Association*, 91: 1,103–7.

Martyn, C. (1989), 'Geographical relation between Alzheimer's disease and aluminium in drinking water', *The Lancet*, 2: 59–62.

Masters, C.L., Harris, J.O., Gajdusek, D.C., Gibbs, C.J. et al. (1970), 'Creutzfeldt-Jakob disease: Patterns of worldwide occurrence and the significance of familial and sporadic clustering', *Annals of Neurology*, 5: 177–88.

Mathuranath P.S., Nestor P.J., Berrios G.E., Rakowicz W. & Hodges J.R. (2000) 'A brief cognitive test battery to differentiate Alzheimer's disease and fronto-temporal dementia'. *Neurology, 55,* 1613-1620.

Mattis, S. (1988a), *Dementia Rating Scale*, Windsor: NFER-Nelson.

Mattis, S. (1988b), 'Mental status examination for organic mental syndrome in the elderly patient', in Bellak, L. & Karasu, T. (eds), *Geriatric Psychiatry: A Handbook for Psychiatrists and Primary Care*

Physicians, New York: Grune & Stratton.

Maugh II, T.H. (1995), 'New drug shows promise against multiple sclerosis', *Los Angeles Times*, 6 February: A19–A20.

May, W.W. (1968), 'Creutzfeldt-Jakob disease', *Acta Neurologica Scandinavica*, 44: 1–32.

Mayes, A.R. (1986), 'Learning and memory disorders and their assessment', *Neuropsychologia*, 24: 25–39.

Mayes, A.R., Meudell, P.R., Mann, D. & Pickering, A. (1988), 'Location of lesions in Korsakoff's syndrome: Neuropsychological and neuropathological data on two patients', *Cortex*, 24: 367–88.

McCue, M., Rogers, J.C. & Goldstein, G. (1990), 'Relationships between neuropsychological and functional assessment in elderly neuropsychiatric patients', *Rehabilitation Psychology*, 35: 91–5.

McDade, H.L. & Adler, S. (1980), 'Down syndrome and short-term memory impairment: A storage or retrieval deficit?' *American Journal of Mental Deficiency*, 84, 6: 561–7.

McDonald, A.J.D. (1986), 'Do general practitioners "miss" depression in elderly patients?', *British Medical Journal*, May, 292: 1,365–7.

McDonald, E. (1992), 'Multiple sclerosis: Common management issues', *Australian Family Physician*, 21, 10: 1,421–4.

McGowin, D.F. (1993), *Living in the Labyrinth: A Personal Journey Through the Maze of Alzheimer's*, San Francisco: Elder Books.

McGrath, S.D. & McKenna, J. (1961), 'The Ganser syndrome: A critical review', *Proceedings of the Third World Congress of Psychiatry*, 1: 156–61.

McKhann, G., Drachman, D. & Folstein, M. (1984), 'Clinical diagnosis of Alzheimer's disease', *Neurology*, 34: 939–44.

McKinlay WW & Brooks N (1984) 'Methodological problems in assessing recovery following severe head injury'. *Journal of Clinical Neuropsychology, 6,* 87-99.

McKusick, V.A. (1983), *Mendelian Inheritance in Man* (6th edn), Baltimore: The Johns Hopkins University Press, 30–1.

McNemar, Q. (1957), 'On WAIS difference scores', *Journal of Consulting Psychology*, 21: 239–40.

Medical Research Council (1987), *Report from the MRC Alzheimer's Disease Workshop*, London: HMSO.

Medical Research Council (1993), 'Recommendations on the dietary management of phenylketonuria', *Archives of Diseases in Childhood*, 68: 426–7.

Mental Health Foundation (1993), *Learning Disabilities: The Fundamental Facts*, London: Mental Health Foundation.

Mikkelsohn, S., Gregersen, P. & Klausen, H. (1978), ('Presenile dementia as an occupational disease following industrial exposure to organic solvent: A review of the literature'), *Ugeskrift for Läeger*,

140: 1,633–8.

Mikkelsohn, S. (1980), 'A cohort study of disability pension and death among painters with special regard to disabling presenile dementia as an occupational disease', *Scandinavian Journal of Social Medicine*, Supplement 16: 34–43.

Miller, A.K.H., Alston, R.L. & Corsellis, J.A.N. (1980), 'Variation with age in the volumes of grey and white matter in the cerebral hemispheres of man: Measurements with an image analyser', *Neuropathology & Applied Neurobiology*, 6: 119–32.

Miller, C.M. (1993), 'Trajectory and empowerment theory applied to care of patients with multiple sclerosis', *Journal of Neuroscience Nursing*, 25, 6: 343–8.

Miller, C.M. & Hens, M. (1993), 'Multiple sclerosis: A literature review', *Journal of Neuroscience Nursing*, 25, 3: 174–9.

Miller, E. (1971), 'On the nature of the memory disorder in presenile dementia', *Neuropsychologia*, 9: 75–81.

Miller, E. (1973), 'Short and long term memory in patients with presenile dementia (Alzheimer's disease)', *Psychological Medicine*, 3: 221–4.

Miller, E. (1975), 'Impaired recall and memory disturbance', *British Journal of Social & Clinical Psychology*, 14: 73–9.

Miller, E. (1977), *Abnormal Ageing: The Psychology of Senile and Presenile Dementia*, London: John Wiley.

Miller, E. (1981), 'The nature of the cognitive deficit in senile dementia', in Miller, N.E. & Cohen, G.D. (eds), *Clinical Aspects of Alzheimer's Disease and Senile Dementia*, New York: Raven Press.

Miller, E. & Morris, R. (1993), *The Psychology of Dementia*, Chichester: John Wiley.

Miniszek, N.A. (1983), 'Development of Alzheimer's disease in Down's syndrome individuals', *American Journal of Mental Deficiency*, 85: 377-385.

Mitrushina, M., Uchiyama, C. & Satz, P. (1995), 'Heterogeneity of cognitive profiles in normal aging: implications for early manifestations of Alzheimer's disease', *Journal of Clinical and Experimental Neuropsychology*, 17; 3: 374-382.

Mohanaruban, K., Sastry, B.S.D. & Finucane, P. (1989), 'Assessment and diagnosis of dementia', *Geriatric Medicine*, June: 81–4.

Money, E.A., Kirk, R.C. & McNaughton, N. (1992), 'Alzheimer's dementia produces a loss of discrimination but no increase in rate of memory decay in delayed matching to sample', *Neuropsychologia*, 30: 133-143.

Moody, P. & Moody, R. (1992), 'Half Left', Oslo: Dreyers Forlag A/S.

Montgomery, G.K. & Erickson, L.M. (1987), 'Neuropsychological perspectives in amyotrophic lateral sclerosis', *Neurology Clinics*, 5:

61–81.

Mori, H., Kondo, J. & Ihara, Y. (1987), 'Ubiquitin is a component of paired helical filaments in Alzheimer's disease', *Science*, 235: 1,641–4.

Morris, J.C. & Fulling, K. (1988), 'Early Alzheimer's disease: Diagnostic considerations', *Archives of Neurology*, 45, 3: 345–9.

Morris, R.G. (1983), 'The effect of concurrent articulation on memory span in Alzheimer-type dementia', *British Journal of Clinical Psychology*, 26: 233–4.

Morris, R.G. (1984), 'Dementia and the functioning of the articulatory loop system', *Cognitive Neuropsychology*, 1: 143–57.

Morris, R.G. (1986), 'Short-term forgetting in senile dementia of the Alzheimer's type', *Cognitive Neuropsychology*, 3: 77–97.

Morris, R.G. (1987a), 'The effect of concurrent articulation on memory span in Alzheimer-type dementia', *British Journal of Clinical Psychology*, 26: 233-234.

Morris, R.G. (1987b), 'Articulatory rehearsal in Alzheimer-type dementia', *Brain & Language, 30:* 351-362.

Morris, R.G. (1992), 'Patterns of Short-Term Memory Impairment in Alzheimer's Disease' in Backman, L. (ed), *Memory Functioning in Dementia*, Amsterdam: Elsevier, 3-25.

Morris, R.G. (1994a), 'Working memory in Alzheimer-type dementia', *Neuropsychology, 8;* 4: 544-554.

Morris, R.G. (1994b), 'Recent developments in the neuropsychology of dementia', *International Review of Psychiatry, 6:* 85-107.

Morris, R.G. & Kopelman, M.D. (1986), 'The memory deficits in Alzheimer-type dementia: A review', *Quarterly Journal of Experimental Psychology*, 38: 575–602.

Morris, R.G. & McKiernan, F. (1993), 'Neuropsychological investigation of dementia', in Burns, A. & Levy, R. (eds), *Dementia*, London: Chapman & Hall.

Morris, R.G., Wheatley, J. & Britton, P.G. (1983), 'Retrieval from long-term memory in senile dementia: Cued recall revisited', *British Journal of Clinical Psychology*, 22: 141–2.

Moss, S., Goldberg, D. & Patel, P. (1991), 'Psychiatric and physical morbidity in older people with severe mental handicap', *Report*, University of Manchester: Hester Adrian Centre.

Moss, S., Hogg, J. & Horne, M. (1992), 'Demographic characteristics of a population of people with moderate, severe and profound intellectual disability (mental handicap) over 50 years of age: Age, structure, IQ and adaptive skills', *Journal of Intellectual Disability Research*, 36: 387–401.

Moulin, L. (1980), 'How reliable are the IQ tests currently in use with the mentally handicapped? A study of the use of two tests (WAIS &

Stanford Binet) on 20 subjects', *Apex, Journal of the British Institute of Mental Handicap*, 8, 2: 45–6.

Muir, W.J., Squire, I. & Blackwood, D.H.R. (1988), 'Auditory P300 response in the assessment of Alzheimer's disease in Down's syndrome: A 2-year follow-up study', *Journal of Mental Deficiency Research*, 32: 455–63.

Mulder, D.W. & Howard, F.M. (1976), 'Patient resistance and prognosis in amyotrophic lateral sclerosis', *Mayo Clinic Proceedings*, 51: 537–41.

Murphy, E. (1982), 'Social origins of depression in old age', *British Journal of Psychiatry*, 141: 135–42.

Murphy, G. & Langley, J. (1995), *Working with Older People: 10 Training Workshops*, Bicester: Winslow Press.

Myrianthopoulos, N.C. (1966), 'Huntington's chorea', *Journal of Medical Genetics*, 3: 298–314.

Naglieri, J.A. (1985), *The Matrix Analogies Test – Expanded Form*, New York: The Psychological Corporation.

Naglieri, J.A. & Das, J.P. (1987), 'Construct and criterion-related validity of planning, simultaneous, and successive cognitive processing tasks', *Journal of Psychoeducational Assessment*, 4: 353–63.

Naglieri, J.A. & Das, J.P. (1988), 'Planning-Arousal-Simultaneous-Successive (PASS): A model for assessment', *Journal of School Psychology*, 26: 35–48.

Nelson, H.E. & Willison, J.R. (1991), *National Adult Reading Test (NART) Test Manual*, 2nd edn, Windsor: NFER-Nelson.

Nerenz, D. & Leventhal, H. (1983), 'Self-regulation theory in chronic illness', in Burish, T. & Bradley, L.A. (Eds), *Coping with Chronic Disease: Research and Applications*, London: Academic Press.

Neugut, R.H., Neugut, A.I., Kahana, E., Stein, Z., et al. (1979), 'Creutzfeldt-Jakob disease: Familial clustering among Libyan-born Israelis', *Neurology*, 29: 225–31.

Nevin, S. (1967), 'On some aspects of cerebral degeneration in later life', *Proceedings of the Royal Society of Medicine*, 60: 517–26.

Nevin, S., McMenemey, W.H., Behram, S. & Jones, D.P. (1960), 'Subacute spongiform encephalopathy – a subacute form of encephalopathy attributable to vascular dysfunction (spongiform cerebral atrophy)', *Brain*, 83: 519–64.

Newens A.J., Forster, G.P. & Kay, D.W.K. (1995) Dependency and community care in pre-senile Alzheimer's disease. *British Journal of Psychiatry, 166,* 777-782.

NHS – National Health Service (2001) *National Service Framework for Older People.* London, Department of Health.

Norman, D.A. & Shallice, T. (1986), 'Reflections on Cognition and

Parallel Distributed Processing' in McClelland, J.L. & Rumelhart, D.E. (eds), *Parallel Distributed Processing: Exploration of the Microstructure of Cognition. Volume 2*, Cambridge, Massechusetts: MIT Press, 102-110.

Nyberg, L., Backman, L., Erngrund, K., Olofsson, U. & Nilsson, L.G. (1996), 'Age differences in episodic memory, semantic memory, and priming: relationships to demographic, intellectual, and biological factors', *Journal of Gerontology, 51;* 4: P234-P40.

Nicolson, N. & Paly, J. (1981), 'What are the principles of practice?' *Community Care*, July: 14.

Norman, A. (1986), *Aspects of Ageism: A Discussion Paper*, London: Centre for Policy on Ageing.

Nussbaum, P.D., Goreczny, A. & Haddad, L. (1995), 'Cognitive correlates of functional capacity in elderly depressed versus patients with probable Alzheimer's disease', *Neuropsychological Rehabilitation*, 5, 4: 333–40.

O'Connor M, Butters N, Miliotis P, Eslinger P & Cermak LS (1992) The dissociation of anterograde and retrograde amnesia in a patient with herpes encephalitis. *Journal of Clinical & Experimental Neuropsychology, 14*, 159-178.

Oliver, C. & Holland, A.J. (1986), 'Down's syndrome and Alzheimer's disease: A review', *Psychological Medicine*, 16: 307–22.

Oliver, J.E. (1970), 'Huntington's chorea in Northamptonshire', *British Journal of Psychiatry*, 116: 241–53.

Olson, M.I. & Shaw, C.M. (1969), 'Presenile dementia and Alzheimer's disease in mongolism', *Brain*, 95: 147–56.

OPCS (Office of Population, Census and Statistics) (1985), *Social Trends*, Fareham: OPCS.

Owen, M., Liddel, M. & McGuffin, P. (1994), 'An association with apolipoprotein E4 may help unlock the puzzle', *British Medical Journal*, 308: 672–3.

Palmer, C.G.S., Crank, C., Pueschel, S.M., Wisniewski, K.E., *et al.*. (1992), 'Head circumference of children with Down's syndrome (0-36 months)', *American Journal of Medical Genetics, 42:* 61-67.

Parkin, A.J. (1991), 'Recent advances in the neuropsychology of memory', in Weinman, J. & Hunter, J. (eds), *Memory: Neurochemical and Abnormal Perspectives*, London: Hardwood.

Parkin, A.J., Walter, B.M. & Hunkin, N.M. (1995), 'Relationships between normal aging, frontal lobe function, and memory for temporal and spatial information', *Neuropsychology, 9;* 3: 304-312.

Parsons, O.A. (1977), 'Neuropsychological deficits in alcoholics: Facts and fancies', *Alcoholism: Clinical & Experimental Research*, 1: 51-6.

Pattie, A. & Gilleard, C. (1979), *Clifton Assessment Procedures for the Elderly*, Windsor: NFER-Nelson.

Penson, J. (1990), *Bereavement: A Guide for Nurses*, London: Chapman & Hall.

Perlick, D. & Atkins, A. (1984), 'Variations in the reported age of a patient: A source of bias in the diagnosis of depression and dementia', *Journal of Consulting and Clinical Psychology*, 52: 812–20.

Perry, G., Friedman, R., Shaw, G. & Chau, V. (1987), 'Ubiquitin is detected in neurofibrillary tangles and senile plaque neurites of Alzheimer's disease brains', *Proceedings of the National Academy of Science (USA)*, 84: 3,033–6.

Peters, P.K., Wendell, M.S. & Mulder, D.W. (1978), 'Is there a characteristic profile in amyotrophic lateral sclerosis? A Minnesota Multiphasic Personality Inventory study', *Archives of Neurology*, 35: 322–33.

Peterson, L.R. & Peterson, M.J. (1959), 'Short-term retention of individual verbal items', *Journal of Experimental Psychology*, 58: 193–8.

Peyser, J.M., Edwards, K.R., Poser, C.M. & Filskov, S.B. (1980), 'Cognitive function in patients with multiple sclerosis', *Archives of Neurology*, 37: 577–9.

Philpot, M.P. & Levy, R. (1987), 'A memory clinic for the early diagnosis of dementia', *International Journal of Geriatric Psychiatry*, 2: 195–200.

Piedmont, R.L., Sokolove, R.L. & Fleming, M.Z. (1989), 'On WAIS-R difference scores in a psychiatric sample', *Psychological Assessment: A Journal of Consulting & Clinical Psychology*, 1: 155–9.

Poirier, J., Davignon, J., Bouthillier, D., Kogan, S., et al. (1993), 'Apolipoprotein E polymorphism and Alzheimer's disease', *The Lancet*, 342: 697–9.

Poser, C.M. (1983), 'New diagnostic criteria for multiple sclerosis: Guidelines for research protocols', *Annals of Neurology*, 13: 227–31.

Powell, T., Brooker, D.J.R. & Papadopolous, A. (1993), 'Test-retest reliability of the Middlesex Assessment of Mental State (MEAMS): A preliminary investigation in people with probable dementia', *British Journal of Clinical Psychology*, 32: 224-226.

Prosser, G. (1989), 'Down's syndrome, Alzheimer's disease, and reality orientation', *Mental Handicap, 17;* 2: 50-53.

Prien, R.F. (1973), 'Chemotherapy in chronic organic brain syndrome – a review of the literature', *Psychopharmacology Bulletin*, 9: 5–20.

Pueschel, S.M., Yeatman, S. & Hum, C. (1977), 'Discontinuing the pheny-lalanine-restricted diet in young children with PKU', *Journal* of the American Dietetic Association, May, 70: 506–9.

Räihä, I., Kaprio, J., Koskenvuo, M., Rajala, T., et al. (1996), 'Alzheimer's disease in Finnish twins', *The Lancet*, 347: 573–8.

Rao, S.M., Hammeke, T.A., McQuillen, M.P., Khatri, O.O., et al. (1984), 'Memory disturbance in chronic progressive multiple sclerosis', *Archives of Neurology*, 41: 625–31.

Rao, S.M., Huber, S.J. & Bornstein, R.A. (1992), 'Emotional changes with multiple sclerosis and Parkinson's disease', *Journal of Consulting & Clinical Psychology*, 60, 3: 369–78.

Ratcliffe, J., Rittman, A., Wolf, S. & Verity, M.A. (1975), 'Creutzfeldt-Jakob disease with focal onset unsuccessfully treated with amantadine', *Bulletin of the Los Angeles Neurological Society*, 40: 18–20.

Rau, M.T. (1993), *Coping with Communication Challenges and Alzheimers*, London: Chapman & Hall. Raven, J., Raven, J.C. & Court, J.H. (1990), *Coloured Progressive Matrices*, Oxford: Oxford Psychologists Press.

Raven, J.C., Court, J.H. & Raven, J. (1995), '*Raven Manual: Section 2. Coloured Progressive Matrices 1995 Edition*', Oxford: Oxford Psychologists Press.

Reding, M., Haycox, J. & Blass, J.P. (1985), 'Depression in patients referred to a dementia clinic', *Archives of Neurology*, 42: 894–6.

Reid, A.H. (1982), *The Psychiatry of Mental Handicap*, London: Blackwell.

Reid, A.H. & Aungle, P.G. (1974), 'Dementia in ageing mentally defectives: A clinical psychiatric study', *Journal of Mental Deficiency Research*, 18: 15–23.

Reid, A.H., Maloney, A.F.J. & Aungle, P.G. (1978), 'Dementia in ageing mentally defectives: A clinical and neuropathological study', *Journal of Mental Deficiency Research*, 22: 233–41.

Reisberg, B. (1983), 'An overview of current concepts of Alzheimer's disease, senile dementia, and age-associated cognitive decline', in Reisberg, B. (ed.), *Alzheimer's Disease, the Standard Reference*, New York: The Free Press.

Reitan, R.M. (1955) The relation of the Trail Making Test to organic brain damage. *Journal of Consulting & Clinical Psychology*, *19*, 393-394.

Reitan, R.M. (1967), 'Psychological changes associated with aging and cerebral damage', *Mayo Clinic Proceedings*, 42: 653–73.

Reitan, R. (1992) *Trail Making Test: Manual for Administration and Scoring.* Tucson: Reitan Psychological Laboratory.

Repp, A.C., Felce, D. & Barton, L.E. (1988), 'Basing the treatment of stereotypic and self-injurious behaviours on hypotheses of their causes', *Journal of Applied Behavior Analysis*, 21, 3: 281–9.

Richardson, J.T.E. (1992), 'Imagery mnemonics and memory remediation', *Neurology*, 42: 283–6.

Robertson-Tchabo, E.A., Hausen, C.P. & Arenberg, D. (1976), 'A classical mnemonic for older learners: A trip that works', *Educational Gerontologist*, 1: 215-16.

Roediger III, H.L. & Blaxton, T.A. (1987), 'Retrieval modes produce dissociations in memory for surface information', in Gosfein, D. & Hoffman, R.R. (eds), *Memory and Cognitive Processes: The Ebbinghaus Centennial Conference*, New Jersey: Lawrence Erlbaum.

Roos, R.P. (1981), 'Alzheimer's disease and the lessons of transmissible virus dementia', in Mortimer, J.A. & Schuman, L.M. (eds), *The Epidemiology of Dementia*, London: Oxford University Press.

Roper, A.H. & Williams, R.S. (1980), 'Relationship between plaques, tangles and dementia in Down's syndrome', *Neurology*, 30: 639–44.

Rosen, W.G., Mohs, R.C. & Davis, K.L. (1984), 'A new rating scale for Alzheimer's disease', *American Journal of Psychiatry*, 141, 11: 1,357–64.

Rosen, W.G., Terry, R.D. & Fuld, P.A. (1980), 'Pathological verification of ischaemic scores in differentiation of dementia', *Annals of Neurology*, 7: 486–8.

Roth, M. (1955), 'The natural history of mental disorders in old age', *Journal of Mental Science*, 102: 281–93.

Roth, M. (1981), 'The diagnosis of dementia in late and middle life', in Mortimer, J.A. & Schuman, L.M. (eds), *The Epidemiology of Dementia*, London: Oxford University Press.

Roth, M., Tym, E. & Mountjoy, C.Q. (1986), 'CAMDEX: a standardised instrument for the diagnosis of mental disorder in the elderly with special reference to the early detection of dementia', *British Journal of Psychiatry*, 149: 698–709.

Royall, D.R. & Mahurin, R.K. (1994), 'Qualitative dementia types', *American Journal of Geriatric Psychiatry*, 2, 2: 178–9.

Russell WR (1971) *The Traumatic Amnesias*. Oxford: Oxford University Press.

Sagar, H.J., Corkin, S., Cohen, N.J. & Growden, J.H. (1984), 'Remote-memory function in Alzheimer's disease and Parkinson's disease', *Brain*, 111: 698–718.

Sahakian, B.J., Morris, R.G., Evenden, J.L., Heald, A., Levy, R., Philpot, M. & Robbins, T.W. (1988), 'A comparative study of visuospatial memory and learning in Alzheimer-type dementia and Parkinson's disease', *Brain, 111:* 698-718.

Sanders, W.L. (1979), 'Creutzfeldt-Jakob disease treated with amantadine', *Journal of Neurology, Neurosurgery & Psychiatry*, 42:

960–1.

Sanders, W.L. & Dunn, T.L. (1973), 'Creutzfeldt-Jakob disease treated with amantadine', *Journal of Neurology, Neurosurgery & Psychiatry*, 36: 581–4.

Saxton J., McGonigle K.L., Swihart A.A. & Boller F. (1993) *Severe Impairment Battery. Manual.* Bury St Edmunds: Thames Valley Test Company.

Schaie, K.W. (1958), 'Rigidity–flexibility and intelligence: A cross-sectional study of the adult life span from 20 to 70 years', *Psychological Monographs*, 72, 9: 462.

Schapiro, M.B., Luxemberg, J.S., Kaye, J.A., Haxby, J.V., et al. (1987), 'Serial quantitative computed tomography analysis of brain morphometry in adult Down's syndrome at different ages', *Annals of Neurology*, 22: 432.

Schellenberg, G.D., Bird, T.D. & Wijsman, E.M. (1992), 'Genetic linkage evidence for a familial Alzheimer's disease locus on chromosome 14', *Science*, 258: 668–71.

Schneck, M.H., Reisberg, B. & Ferris, S.H. (1982), 'An overview of current concepts of Alzheimer's disease', *American Journal of Psychiatry*, 139: 165–73.

Schumacher, G.A. (1965), 'Problems of experimental trials of therapy in multiple sclerosis: report by the panel on the evaluation of experimental trials of therapy in multiple sclerosis', *Annals of the New York Academy of Science*, 122: 552–68.

Scott, P.D. (1965), 'The Ganser syndrome', *British Journal of Criminology*, 5: 127–31.

Seguin, E. (1866), *Idiocy: Its Treatment by the Physiological Method*, New York: William Wood.

Seligman, M.E.P. (1975), *Helplessness*, San Francisco: Freeman.

Seltzer, M. & Krauss, M. (1987), *Aging and Mental Retardation: Extending the Continuum*, Washington, DC: American Association on Mental Deficiency.

Shallice, T. (1988), *'From Neuropsychology to Mental Structure'*, New York: Cambridge University Press.

Shapiro, M.B., Haxby, J.V., Grady, C.L. (1992), 'The nature of mental retardation and dementia in Down's syndrome: Study with PET, CT and neuropsychology', *Neurobiology of Ageing*, 13: 723–4.

Shapiro, M.B., Haxby, J.V., Grady, C.L. & Raroport, S.I. (1986), 'Cerebral glucose utilization, quantitative tomography, and cognitive function in adult Down syndrome', in Epstein, C.J. (ed.), *The Neurobiology of Down Syndrome*, New York: Raven.

Shermann, S.L., Takesu, N., Freeman, S.B., Grantham, M., et al. (1991), 'Association between reduced recombination with nondisjunction', *American Journal of Human Genetics*, 49: 608–

20.

Shuttleworth, E.C., Huber, S.J. & Paulson, G.W. (1987), 'Depression in patients with dementia of Alzheimer's type', *Journal of the National Medical Association*, 79: 733–6.

Singh DNP & Cookson FB (1983) *Atlas of the Human Brain and Spinal Cord*. Beckenham: Croom Helm, 4; 8.

Sluss, T.K., Gruenberg, E.M. & Kramer, M. (1981), 'The use of longitudinal studies in the investigation of risk factors for senile dementia of Alzheimer type', in Mortimer, J.A. & Schuman, L.M. (eds), *The Epidemiology of Dementia*, New York: Oxford University Press.

Solitaire, G.B. & Lamarche, J.B. (1966), 'Alzheimer's disease and senile dementia as seen in mongoloids: Neuropathological observations', *American Journal of Mental Deficiency*, 70: 840–8. Somerset County Council (1992), *Care in the Community: Strategy for Persons in Mental Handicap Hospitals*, Taunton: Somerset County Council.

Sourander, P. & Sjögren, H. (1970), 'The concept of Alzheimer's disease and its related implications', in Wolstenholme, G.E.W. & O'Connor, M. (eds), *CIBA Foundation Symposium: AD and Related Conditions*, London: Churchill, 11–36.

Spinnler, H. & Della Sala, S. (1988), 'The role of clinical neuropsychology in the neurological diagnosis of Alzheimer's disease', *Journal of Neurology*, 235: 258-271.

Spinnler, H., Della Sala, S., Bandera, R. & Baddeley, A. (1988), 'Dementia, ageing, and the structure of human memory', *Cognitive Neuropsychology*, 5: 193–211.

Spreen, O. & Strauss, E. (1991), *A Compendium of Neuropsychological Tests: Administration, Norms and Commentary*, New York: Oxford University Press.

Squire, L.R. (1974), 'Remote memory as affected by aging', *Neuropsychologia*, 12: 429–35.

Squire, L.R. (1992), 'Memory and the hippocampus: A synthesis from findings with rats, monkeys, and humans', *Psychological Review*, 99: 195–231.

St Clair, D.M. & Blackwood, D.H. (1985), 'Premature senility in Down's syndrome', *The Lancet*, 2: 34.

St George-Hyslop, P.H., Tanzi, R.E., Polinsky, R.J., Haines, J.L., et al. (1987), 'The genetic defect causing familial Alzheimer's disease maps on chromosome 21', *Science*, 235: 885–90.

Steingart, A., Hachinski, V.C., Lay, C. & Fox, A.J. (1987), 'Cognitive and neurologic findings in demented patients with diffuse white matter lucencies on computed tomographic scan (leuko-araiosis)', *Archives of Neurology*, 44, 1: 36–9.

Stokes, G. (1995), *On Being Old – The Psychology of Later Life*,

Brighton: Falmer Press.

Stokes, G. & Holden, U. (1993), 'Dementia: Causes and clinical syndromes', in Stokes, G. & Goudie, F. (eds), *Working with Dementia*, Bicester: Winslow Press.

Struwe, F (1929), 'Histopathologische Untersuchungen über Entstehung und Wesen der senilen Plaques' ('Hisopathological investigations concerning the formation and existence of senile plaques'), *Zeitshrift für die gesamte Neurologie und Psychiatrie*, 122: 291.

Sullivan, E.V., Corkin, S. & Growden, J.H. (1986), 'Verbal and non-verbal short-term memory in patients with Alzheimer's disease and in healthy elderly subjects', *Developmental Neuropsychology*, 2: 387–400.

Swash, M., Brooks, D.N., Day, N.E., Frith, C.D., et al. (1991), 'Clinical trials in Alzheimer's disease', *Journal of Neurology, Neurosurgery & Psychiatry*, 54: 178–81.

Swearer, J.M. & Kane, K.J. (1996), 'Behavioral slowing with age: boundary conditions of the generalized slowing model', *Journal of Gerontology, 51:* 4: P189-P200.

Sylvester, P.E. (1984), 'Ageing in the mentally retarded', in Dobbing, J., Clarke, A.D.B., Corbett, J.A., Hogg, J. & Robinson, R.O. (eds), *Scientific Studies in Mental Retardation*, London: Royal Society of Medicine/ Macmillan.

Talland, G.A. (1965), *Deranged Memory*, New York: Academic Press.

Tangye, S.R. (1979), 'The EEG and incidence of epilepsy in Down's syndrome', *Journal of Mental Deficiency Research*, 23: 17–24.

Tarter, R.E. & Jones, B.M. (1971), 'Absence of intellectual deterioration in chronic alcoholics', *Journal of Clinical Psychology*, 27: 453–4.

Terr, L. (1994), *Unchained Memories: True Stories of Traumatic Memories, Lost and Found*, London: Basic Books.

Terry, R. & Pena, C. (1965), 'Experimental production of neurofibrillary degeneration', *Journal of Neuropathology and Experimental Neurology*, 24: 200–10.

Thase, M.E. (1982), 'Reversible dementia in Down's syndrome', *Journal of Mental Deficiency Research*, 26: 111–13.

Thase, M.E., Tigner, R., Smeltzer, D.J. & Liss, L. (1983), 'Age-related neuropsychological deficits in Down's syndrome', *Biological Psychiatry*, 19, 4: 571–85.

Thomas, J.C., Fozard, J.L. & Waugh, N.C. (1977), 'Age-related differences in naming latency', *American Journal of Psychology*, 90: 499–509.

Thompson D (Ed) (1995t) *The Concise Oxford English Dictionary.* 9th Ed'n. Oxford: Oxford University Press, 850.

Thompson, L.W., Davis, G.C., Obrist, W.D. & Heyman, A. (1976),

'Effects of hyperbaric oxygen on behavioral and physiological measures in elderly demented patients', *Journal of Gerontology*, 31: 23–8.

Thompson, S.B.N. (1989), 'Techniques for tackling anxiety', *Therapy Weekly*, 15, 49: 6.

Thompson, S.B.N. (1990), 'Talking about sex . . .', *Therapy Weekly*, 17, 13: 8.

Thompson, S.B.N. (1992), 'Traitement de la dépression en rééducation cardiague ambulatoire' ('Treatment of depression in the rehabilitation of cardiac outpatients'), *Visages de la Dépression*, March: 9–10.

Thompson SBN (1993) *Eating Disorders: A Guide for Health Professionals.* London: Chapman & Hall.

Thompson, S.B.N. (1993a), 'Down's syndrome and Alzheimer's disease', *Therapy Weekly*, 19, 21: 8.

Thompson, S.B.N. (1993b), *Eating Disorders: A Guide for Health Professionals*, London: Chapman & Hall.

Thompson, S.B.N. (1994a), 'A neuropsychological test battery for identifying dementia in people with learning disabilities', *British Journal of Developmental Disabilities*, 40, 2(79): 135–42.

Thompson, S.B.N. (1994b), 'Sexuality training in occupational therapy for people with learning disability, four years on: Policy guidelines', *British Journal of Occupational Therapy*, 57, 7: 255–8.

Thompson, S.B.N. (1995a), 'Storage problems', *Therapy Weekly*, 21, 40: 7.

Thompson, S.B.N. (1995b), 'Observed behaviour of a woman with a childhood diagnosis of phenylketonuria and a profound learning disability', *British Journal of Developmental Disabilities*, 40, 2(79): 135–42.

Thompson, S.B.N. (1996a), 'Providing a neuropsychology service for people with multiple sclerosis in an interdisciplinary rehabilitation unit', *Disability & Rehabilitation*, 18, 7: 348–53.

Thompson, S.B.N. (1996b), 'Practical ways of improving memory storage and retrieval problems in patients with head injuries', *British Journal of Occupational Therapy*, 59, 9: 418–22.

Thompson, S.B.N. (1997) *Dementia: A Guide for Health Care Professionals.* Aldershot: Arena.

Thompson SBN (2002) 'Memory decline, Alzheimer's disease and vascular dementia: The clinical picture'. *Journal of Cognitive Rehabilitation, 20;* 2: 12-18.

Thompson, S.B.N. (2003) *Memory Problems: A Self-Help Guide for Patients, Carers, Health Care Professionals and Students in Training.* Chichester: Oxford Press.

Thompson SBN, MacDonald J & Coates TD (2001) 'Improving visual memory with Aricept (Donepezil Hydrochloride, E2020) in mild-tomoderate Alzheimer's disease'. *Clinical Gerontologist, 24* (1/2); 12, 55-73.

Thompson, S.B.N. & Martin, S. (1993), 'The pleasure of plasma', *Therapy Weekly*, 20, 13: 17.

Thompson, S.B.N. & Martin, S. (1994), 'Making sense of multi-sensory rooms for people with learning disabilities', *British Journal of Occupational Therapy*, 57, 9: 341–4.

Thompson, S.B.N. & Morgan, M. (1996), *Occupational Therapy for Stroke Rehabilitation* (2nd reprint), London: Chapman & Hall.

Thompson, S.B.N., North, N. & Pentland, B. (1992), 'Clinical management of a man with complex partial seizures and a severe head injury', *Brain Injury*, 7, 3: 257–62.

Thompson SBN & Watson F (2001) 'Hollywood *Wives*': Education and support for spouses of inpatients with dementia. *Journal of Dementia Care, 9;* 2: 38.

Tierney, M., Fisher, R. & Lewis, A.J. (1988), 'The NINCDS/ADRDA Work Group criteria for the clinical diagnosis of probable Alzheimer's disease: A clinicopathologic study of 57 cases', *Neurology*, 37: 359–64.

Tomlinson, B.E., Blessed, G. & Roth, M. (1970), 'Observations on the brains of demented old people', *Journal of the Neurological Sciences*, 11: 205–42.

Tout, K. (1993), *Elderly Care: A World Perspective*, London: Chapman & Hall.

Trenerry, M.R., Crosson, B., DeBoe, J. & Leber, W.R. (1989), *Stroop Neuropsychological Screening Test Manual*, Odessa, Florida: Psychological Assessment Resources, Inc.

Tulving, E. (1979), 'Relations between encoding specificity and levels of processing', in Cermak, L.S. & Craik, F.I.M. (eds), *Levels of Processing in Human Memory*, New Jersey: Lawrence Erlbaum.

Tulving, E. (1983), *Elements of Episodic Memory*, New York: Oxford University Press.

Tuokko, H. & Crockett, D. (1989), 'Cued recall and memory disorders in dementia', *Journal of Clinical & Experimental Neuropsychology*, 11: 278–94.

Turek, I., Kurland, A.A., Ota, K.Y. & Hanlon, T.E. (1969), 'Effects of pipradol hydrochloride on geriatric patients', *Journal of the American Geriatric Society*, 17: 408–13.

Turnbull, J. (1993), 'Diverse options', *Nursing Times*, 89, 22: 62–3. Vallar, G. & Baddeley, A.D. (1984), 'Fractionation of working memory: Neuropsychological evidence for a phonological short-term store', *Journal of Verbal Learning and Verbal Behavior*, 34: 53–60.

van Belle, G., Uhlmann, R.F., Hughes, J.P. & Larson. E.B. (1990), 'Reliability of estimates of change in mental status test performance in senile dementia of the Alzheimer type', *Journal of Clinical Epidemiology, 43;* 6: 589-595.

Van Duijn, C.M., Clayton, D.G. & Chandra, V. (1994), 'Interaction between genetic and environmental risk factors for Alzheimer's disease: A reanalysis of case-control studies', *Genetics & Epidemiology*, 11: 539–51.

Vanderplate, C. (1984), 'Psychological aspects of multiple sclerosis and its treatment: Towards a bio-psychosocial perspective', *Health Psychology*, 3: 253–72.

Veall, R.M. (1974), 'The prevalence of epilepsy among mongols related to age', *Journal of Mental Deficiency Research*, 19: 99–106.

Verhaart, W.J.C. & Jelgersma, H.C. (1952), 'Early senile dementia in mongolian idiocy: Description of a case', *Folia Psychiatrica Nederlandica*, 55: 453–9.

Vessie, R.P. (1932), 'On the transmission of Huntington's chorea for 300 years – the Bures family group', *Journal of Nervous & Mental Disease*, 76: 553–73.

Villa, J.L. & Ciompi, L. (1968), 'Therapeutic problems in senile dementia', in Müller, C. & Ciompi, L. (eds), *Senile Dementia: Clinical and Therapeutic Aspects*, Berne: Hans Huber.

Wade, J.P.H., Mirsen, T.R. & Hachinski, V.C. (1987), 'The clinical diagnosis of Alzheimer's disease', *Archives of Neurology*, 44: 24–9. Wainwright, P., Fergusson, R. & Martin, E. (Eds) (1984), *Pocket Dictionary for Nurses*, Oxford: Oxford University Press.

Walton, J.N. (1977), *Brain's Diseases of the Nervous System* (8th edn), Oxford: Oxford University Press.

Warren, A.C., Holroyd, S. & Folstein, M.F. (1989), 'Major depression in Down's syndrome', *British Journal of Psychiatry*, 155: 202–5.

Warrington E (1984) *Recognition Memory Test Manual.* Windsor: NFER-NELSON.

Warrington, E.K. & Weiskrantz, L. (1970), 'Amnesic syndrome: Consolidation or retrieval?' *Nature*, 228: 628–30.

Wassem, R. (1991), 'A test of the relationship between health locus of control and the course of multiple sclerosis', *Rehabilitation Nursing*, 16, 4: 189–93.

Wattis, J. & Church, M. (1986), *Practical Psychiatry of Old Age*, Beckenham: Croom Helm.

Wattis, J. & Martin, C. (1993), *Practical Psychiatry of Old Age*, London: Chapman & Hall.

Wechsler, D. (1955), *Manual for the Wechsler Adult Intelligence Scale*, New York: The Psychological Corporation.

Wechsler, D. (1981a), *Manual for the Wechsler Adult Intelligence Scale*

– *Revised*, New York: The Psychological Corporation.

Wechsler, D. (1981b), *Wechsler Memory Scale – Revised*, San Antonio: Harcourt, Brace, Jovanovich.

Wechsler D (1987) *Wechsler Memory Scale - Revised Manual*. San Antonio: Harcourt, Brace, Jovanovich.

Wechsler, D. (1988). *Wechsler Memory Scale Revised*. San Antonio, Harcourt Brace Jovanovich.

Weisblatt, S.A. (1992), 'Aging in mental retardation', *Current Opinion in Psychiatry*, 5: 664–7.

Welford, A.T. (1977), 'Motor Performance' in Birren, J.E. & Schaie, K.W. (eds), *Handbook of the Psychology of Aging*, New York: Van Nostrand.

Welsh Office (1983), *All Wales Strategy for the Development of Services for Mentally Handicapped People*, Cardiff: HMSO.

Whalley, L.J., Carothers, A.D., Collyer, S., De May, R., et al. (1982), 'A study of familial factors in Alzheimer's disease', *British Journal of Psychiatry*, 140: 49–56. Whitehouse, P.J., Price, D.L., Clark, A.W., Coyle, J.T., et al. (1981), 'Alzheimer's disease: Evidence for selective loss of cholinergic neurons in the nucleus basalis', *Annals of Neurology*, 10: 122–6.

Whitlock, F.A. (1967), 'The Ganser syndrome', *British Journal of Psychiatry*, 113: 19–29.

WHO - World Health Organisation (1992) *The ICD-10 Classification of Mental and Behavioural Disorders*. Geneva: World Health Organisation.

Wilcock, G.K., Hope, R.A., Brooks, D.N. & Lantos, P.L. (1989), 'Recommended minimun data to be collected in research studies on Alzheimer's disease', *Journal of Neurology, Neurosurgery & Psychiatry*, 52: 693–700.

Will, R.G. & Matthews, W.B. (1982), 'Evidence for case-to-case transmission of Creutzfeldt-Jakob disease', *Journal of Neurology, Neurosurgery & Psychiatry*, 45: 235–8.

Willcocks, S. (1994), 'Snoezelen in elderly care', conference report, *British Journal of Occupational Therapy*, 57, 6: 242.

Williams, M. (1970), 'Geriatric patients', in Mittler, P. (ed.), *The Psychological Assessment of Mental and Physical Handicaps*, London: Methuen.

Wilson, B.A. (1992), 'Recovery and compensatory strategies in head injured memory impaired people several years after insult', *Journal of Neurology, Neurosurgery & Psychiatry*, 55: 117–80.

Wilson, B.A., Alderman, N., Burgess, P., Emslie. & Evans, J.J. (1996), '*Behavioural Assessment of the Dysexecutive Syndrome Manual*', Bury St Edmunds: Thames Valley Test Co.

Wilson, B.A. & Baddeley, A.D. (1988), 'Semantic, episodic and autobiographical memory in a postmeningitic patient,' *Brain and Cognition*, 8: 31–46.

Wilson, B.A., Cockburn, J. & Baddeley, A. (1991), *Rivermead Behavioural Memory Test Manual* (2nd edn), Bury St Edmunds: Thames Valley Test Co.

Wilson, B.A. & Moffat, N. (1992), *Clinical Management of Behavioural Problems*, London: Chapman & Hall.

Wilson, R.S., Bacon, L.D., Fox, J.H. & Kaszniak, A.W. (1983), 'Primary memory and secondary memory in dementia of the Alzheimer type', *Journal of Gerontology*, 5: 337–44.

Wineman N.M., O'Brien, R.A., Nealon, N.R. & Kaskel, B. (1993), 'Congruence in uncertainty between individuals with multiple sclerosis and their spouses', *Journal of Neuroscience Nursing*, 25, 6: 356–61.

Wing, L. (1981), 'Asperger's syndrome: A clinical account', *Psychological Medicine*, 11: 115–29.

Wisniewski, K.E., French, J.H., Rosen, L.J., Koziowski, P.B., *et al.* (1983), 'Basal ganglia calcification in Down's syndrome - another manifestation of premature ageing', *Annals of the New York Academy of Sciences, 396*: 179-189.

Wisniewski, K.E., Howe, J., Williams, D.G. & Wisniewski, H.M. (1978), 'Precocious ageing and dementia in patients with Down's syndrome', *Biological Psychiatry*, 13: 619–27.

Wisniewski, K.E. & Rabe, A. (1986), 'Discrepancy between Alzheimer type neuropathology and dementia in persons with Down's syndrome', *Annals of the New York Academy of Sciences*, 477: 247–60.

Wisniewski, K.E., Wisniewski, H.M. & Wen, G.Y. (1985), 'Occurrence of neuropathological changes and dementia of Alzheimer's disease in Down's syndrome', *Annals of Neurology*, 17: 278–82.

Wolf, L.C. & Wright, R.E. (1987), 'Changes in life expectancy of mentally retarded persons in Canadian institutions: A 12 year comparison', *Journal of Mental Deficiency Research*, 31: 41–59.

Wolfensberger, W. & Kugel, R. (1969), *Changing Patterns in Residential Services for the Mentally Retarded*, Washington, DC: President's Committee on Mental Retardation.

Woods, R.T. & Britton, P.G. (1977), 'Psychological approaches to the treatment of the elderly', *Age & Ageing*, 6: 104–12.

Woods, R.T. & Britton, P.G. (1985), *Clinical Psychology With the Elderly*, London: Croom Helm.

Wright, N. & Lindesay, J. (1995) 'A survey of memory clinics in the British Isles'. *International Journal of Geriatric Psychiatry, 10*, 379-385.

Yamauchi, H., Fukuyama, H., Harada, K., Nabatame, H., et al. (1993),

'Callosal atrophy parallels decreased cortical oxygen metabolism and neuropsychological impairment in Alzheimer's disease', *Archives of Neurology*, 50: 1,070–4.

Yapa, P. & Roy, A. (1990), 'Depressive illness and mental handicap: Two case reports', *Mental Handicap*, 18, 1: 19–21.

Yesavage, J.A., Brink, T.L., Rose, T.L., Lum, D., et al. (1983), 'Development and screening of a geriatric depression rating scale: A preliminary report', *Journal of Psychiatric Research*, 7: 37–49.

Yesavage, J.A., Rose, T.L. & Bower, G.H. (1983), 'Interactive imagery and affective judgements improve face-name learning', *Journal of Gerontology*, 38, 2: 198–203.

Young, E.C. & Kramer, B.M. (1991), 'Characteristics of age-related language decline in adults with Down's syndrome', *Mental Retardation*, 29, 2: 75–9.

Zarit, S.H. (1980), *Ageing and Mental Disorders: Psychological Approaches to Assessment and Treatment*, New York: The Free Press.

Zatz, L.M., Jernigan, T.L. & Ahumada, A.J., Jr (1982a), 'Changes on computed cranial tomography with aging: Intracranial fluid volume', *American Journal of Neuroradiology*, 3: 1–11.

Zatz, L.M., Jernigan, T.L. & Ahumada, A.J., Jr (1982b), 'White matter changes in cerebral computed tomography related to aging', *Journal of Computer Assisted Tomography*, 6: 19–23.

Zigman, W.B., Schupf, N., Lubin, R.A. & Silverman, W.P. (1987), 'Premature regression of adults with Down's syndrome', *American Journal of Mental Deficiency*, 92, 2: 161–8.

Zigmond, A.S. & Snaith, R.P. (1983), 'The Hospital Anxiety and Depression Scale', *Acta Psychiatrica Scandinavica*, 67: 361–70.

Index

A-B-C chart 97
Abstract thinking 6
Abulia 5, 24, 96, 183
Acetylcholine esterase inhibitor
    (ACI) 55-56, 108-109
    see also Drugs
Ageing 3-9, 15, 119
    arithmetic ability 5, 89
    normal memory 3, 4, 6, 8-9,
    53-54
    personality change 5
    physical problems 7–8
    posture 5
    psychological problems 7–8
    sexuality 5
    speech 5
    structural changes in brain 5
Ageism 15–17
Agnosia 19, 32, 55
Alcohol problems 48
    see also Korsakoff's psychosis
Alzheimer's disease 20-31, 117-118
    Alois Alzheimer 20
    amyloid precursor protein 26,
    165
    apolipoprotein 26
    attentional impairment 25,
    169
    auditory event-related poten-
    tials 3
    chromosome 19 gene 165,
    166
    drug trials 108-109, 117-118
    heredity 26, 59, 165-166
    management 111-115
    ubiquitin 14
    working memory 118-121
    see also Learning disability
Amnesia
    anterograde 55
    fugue state 55
    post-traumatic 55

retrograde 55
    transient epileptic 54
    see also Head injury
Amygdala 24
Amyotrophic lateral sclerosis 42
Anti-dementia drug
    see Drugs
Anxiety 14, 15, 24, 40, 88, 112,
    135-138
Aphasia 19
Apraxia 19
Aricept (Donepezil Hydrochloride
    E2020) 56, 108
    see also Drugs
Arteriosclerotic dementia 35
Attention 25, 169
    selective 27, 169
    sustained 28
Auditory event-related potentials 3
    see also Alzheimer's disease

Bereavement 109
    Binswanger's disease 35
    see also Dementia
    Bovine spongiform encepha-
    lopathy (BSE)
    see Creutzfeldt-Jakob disease

Ceiling effect 3
    see also Learning disability
    Cerebrovascular accident
    see Stroke
Choreoform
    see Huntington's disease
Chromosome 14 gene 165, 166
Chromosome 19 gene 165, 166
Chromosome 21 gene 58, 165, 166
CJD
    see Creutzfeldt-Jakob disease
Cognitive
    abulia 5, 96, 183
    therapy 7, 107

Computerised tomography 19, 21, 61, 84, 102, 125
   see also Magnetic resonance imaging
Confusion 7
   see also Delirium tremens
Constructional difficulty 19
Creutzfeldt-Jakob disease 39-41, 108
   Bovine spongiform encephalopathy (BSE) 39-40
   kuru 39
   new variant 40-41
   prion 40
   scrapie 39

Delirium tremens 49
   confusion 21, 25
Dementia 3-17, 128
   central executive syndrome 143-160
   chromosome 14 gene 165, 166
   chromosome 19 gene 165, 166
   clinics 122-126
   Creutzfeldt-Jacob disease 39-41
   differential diagnosis 50-52, 158-159
   frontal lobe 30, 35, 49, 53, 147, 148, 168
   habit forming drugs and toxins 50
   heredity 26, 59, 165-166
   Huntington's disease 37-39, 51, 91
   Korsakoff's psychosis 48-49
   lewy body 20, 209
   management 111-115
   Multiple sclerosis 22, 41-42
   Parkinson's disease 36-37, 51
   Pick's disease 35-36, 122
   pseudodementia 44-48
   pugilistica 43-44
   punch drunk syndrome 43
   sexuality 5, 62
   subcortical rteriosclerotic cephalopathy 35
   ubiquitin 14
   vascular 31-34, 61

   see also Depression
   see also Drugs
   see also Learning disability
   see also Memory
Demyelination 41
   see also Multiple sclerosis
Depression 7, 8, 10, 40, 44, 47-48, 51, 88, 91, 107, 112, 135-138
   see also eudodementia
Differential diagnosis 50-52, 158-159
Disorientation 21, 24
   reality orientation 109-110
Donepezil Hydrochloride E2020 (Aricept) 56, 108
   see also Drugs
Down's syndrome 57-59, 127-141
   Alzheimer's disease 57-59
   chromosome 21 gene 58, 165, 166
   Langdon Down 58
   Seguin 58
   trisomy 58, 165
   see also Dementia
   see also Learning disability
Drugs
   acetylcholine esterase inhibitor (ACI) 55-56, 108-109
   Alzheimer's disease 55-56, 107, 166-167
   Aricept (Donepezil Hydrochloride E2020) 56, 108
   Ebixa (Memantine) 109
   Exelon (Rivastigmine Tartrate) 56, 109
   habit-forming 50
   management of dementia 107-109
   Reminyl (Galantamine Hydrobromide) 56, 109
   toxins 50
DSM-III-R 19
DSM-IV 19
Dysexecutive syndrome 148
   see also Dementia

Ebixa (Memantine) 109
   see also Drugs
Encephalopathy 35, 39-40

see also Creutzfeldt-Jakob disease
Exelon (Rivastigmine Tartrate) 56,
    109
  see also Drugs

Fischer plaque 20
Floor effect 3
  see also Learning disability
Free floating anxiety 14
  see also Anxiety
Frontal lobe 30, 35, 49, 53, 147,
    148, 168

Galantamine Hydrobromide (Remi-
    nyl) 56, 109
  see also Drugs
Ganser syndrome 44-45
  see also seudodementia

Haemorrhage 7
  see also Stroke
Hallucination 15
Head injury 53, 54, 75
  see also Amnesia
Hippocampus 24
Huntington's disease 37-39, 51, 91
Hyperspecific learning 94
Hypomania 47
  see also Pseudodementia
Hysterical pseudodementia 45-46
  see also Pseudodementia

Klüver-Bucy syndrome 36
Korsakoff's psychosis 48-49
    vitamin B₁ (thiamine) 33
    Kuru 39
  see also Creutzfeldt-Jakob dis-
    ease

Laevodopa (L-dopa) 37
  see also Parkinson's disease
Language abilities 12, 103
    verbal skills 12
Learning disability 57-65
    Alzheimer's disease 57-59,
    127, 160
    ceiling effect 3
    definition 57
    difficulties in identification

59-61
Down's syndrome 57-59, 127-
    141, 149, 165
floor effect 3
local based hospital units
    (LBHU) 62
multi-sensory room 112
europsychological test battery
    128-129, 148-149
pheylketonuria 64
sexuality 62
social role valorization 61
Snoozelen 112
social, cultural differences
    61-63
Lewy body 20, 209

Mad cow's disease
  see Creutzfeldt-Jakob disease
Magnetic resononance imaging 19,
    21, 84, 102
  see also Computerised tomography
Marijuana 50
  see also Dementia
Memantine (Ebixa) 109
  see also Drugs
Memory
    abnormal 54-56
    age-related 4
    aids 70-71
    anterograde 55
    autobiographical 79
    central executive system 118-
    119, 141-160
    clinics 83-88
    declarative 9, 11, 69
    disorders 54-56
    encoding 8
    episodic 9, 11
    long-term 11, 19
    mammilliary body 170
    normal 53-54
    procedural 9, 11
    registration 8
    retrieval 8, 9
    retrograde 55
    selective 9, 54

semantic 9, 11, 120
short-term/immediate 11, 19
storage 8
strategies 71-77
visual 70, 71, 72, 73-76, 81, 87, 109, 115
visuospatial 30, 108
working 13
see also Dementia
Mental handicap
see Learning disability
Mental imagery
see also Memory (visual)
Miliary plaque 20
Mongolism
see Down's syndrome
Motor neurone disease 42-43
Multi-infarct 20, 22, 61
see also Vascular dementia
Multiple sclerosis 22, 41-42
demyelination 41
optic neuritis 41

Neuritic plaque 20
Neurofibrillary tangle 21
Neuropsychological test battery 128-129, 148-149
ceiling effect 3
floor effect 3

Occupational therapy
see Stroke
Optic neuritis 41
see also Multiple sclerosis

Paraphrenia 14
Parenchymatous senile dementia 20
see also Dementia
Parkinson's disease 36-37, 51
laevodopa (L-dopa) 37
see also Dementia
Personality change 19, 167
see also Ageing
Phenylketonuria 64
see also Learning disability
Phineas Gage 53
see also Head injury
Pick's disease 35-36, 122
see also Dementia

Prejudice 15-17, 63-64
see also Learning disability
Presenile dementia 20
see also Dementia
Primary dementia 19
see also Dementia
Prion 40
see also Creutzfeldt-Jakob disease
Progressive muscle relaxation
see Relaxation
Pseudodementia 44-48
depressive 47-48
see also Dementia
see also Depression

Reality orientation 109-110
see also Disorientation
Relaxation 112-115
mental imagery 115
see also Memory (visual)
Reminyl (Galantamine Hydrobromide) 56, 109
see also Drugs
Rivastigmine Tartrate (Exelon) 56, 109
see also Drugs

Schizophrenia 14, 22, 48
Scrapie 39
see also Creutzfeldt-Jakob disease
Senile dementia 20
see also Dementia
Senile plaque 20-21, 26
Simulated dementia 46-47
see also Pseudodementia
Single assessment process 125
Snoozelen 112
see also Learning disability
Stroke 7, 17, 20, 31
lacunar 20
occupational therapy 17
Thompson digital switch 17
transient ischaemic attack (TIA) 7, 31
Subcortical arterosclerotic encephalopathy 35
see also Dementia

Temporal lobe 24
Thiamine 49
    see also Korsakoff's psychosis
Thompson digital switch 17
TIA (transient ischaemic attack) 31
    see also Stroke
Toxins 50
    see also Drugs
Transient ischaemic attack (TIA) 7,
        31
    see also Stroke
Trisomy 58
    see also Down's syndrome

Ubiquitin 14
    see also Alzheimer's disease

Vascular dementia 31-34, 61
    see also Dementia
Vitamin B$_1$ (thiamine) 49
    see also Korsakoff's psychosis